The
Takeover

The Takeover

An Unexpected Caregiver's Story

Mimi Pockross

Copyright © 2014 by Mimi Pockross.

ISBN: Softcover   978-1-4990-0978-1
           eBook   978-1-4990-0979-8

All rights reserved. No part of this book may be reproduced or transmitted in any form or by any means, electronic or mechanical, including photocopying, recording, or by any information storage and retrieval system, without permission in writing from the copyright owner.

Any people depicted in stock imagery provided by Thinkstock are models, and such images are being used for illustrative purposes only. Certain stock imagery © Thinkstock.

This book was printed in the United States of America.

Rev. date: 09/08/2014

To order additional copies of this book, contact:
Xlibris LLC
1-888-795-4274
www.Xlibris.com
Orders@Xlibris.com
552014

Life is a Journey

    Birth is a beginning and death a destination; But life is a journey. A going, a growing from stage to stage: From childhood to maturity and youth to old age.
    From innocence to awareness and ignorance to knowing; From foolishness to discretion and then perhaps, to wisdom. From weakness to strength or strength to weakness and often back again. From health to sickness and back we pray, to health again.
    From offense to forgiveness, from loneliness to love, From joy to gratitude, from pain to compassion. From grief to understanding, from fear to faith; From defeat to defeat-to-defeat, until, looking backward or ahead:
    We see that victory lies not at some high place along the way, But in having made the journey, stage by stage, a sacred pilgrimage. Birth is a beginning and death a destination; But life is a journey, a sacred pilgrimage, and made stage by stage . . . to life everlasting.

Alvin Fine, 1991

Table of Contents

Dedication 9

Preface 11

Chapter One
    The Beginning 13

Chapter Two
    How Did We Get Here? 21

Chapter Three
    Chicago 31

Chapter Four
    Taking Stock 37

Chapter Five
    Plan B: How About Denver? 43

Chapter Six
    Search II: Denver 47

Chapter Seven
    Moving 53

Chapter Eight
    Settling In 63

Chapter Nine
    Mom's World 75

Chapter Ten
    Life With Dad 87

Chapter Eleven
    Mimi's Daily Drill: Musings from Mimi's Blog and Journals 99

Chapter Twelve
  Celebrating the Holidays 111

Chapter Thirteen
  Going Downhill 115

Chapter Fourteen
  Dad Goes to Respite Care 121

Chapter Fifteen
  Hiring a Care Manager 127

Chapter Sixteen
  Dad Moves to Assisted Living 135

Chapter Seventeen
  Hospice for All 141

Chapter Eighteen
  We Lose Mom 149

Chapter Nineteen
  Dad's Last Days 155

Chapter Twenty
  The Memorial 163

Chapter Twenty-One
  Mourning 169

Chapter Twenty-Two
  Reflections 173

Acknowledgments 179

Appendix I
  Mimi's Ten Commandments Of Eldercare 181

Appendix II
  An Eldercare Primer 185

Appendix III
  Resources 203

Dedication

I moved my 90 and 95 year old mom and dad from Chicago to be with me in Denver in 2011. They both passed away in 2012.

This story of their last year is dedicated to them and to everyone who will experience this journey for others and for themselves.

Preface

This book is the book I wish I could have read when I began the difficult task of caregiving for both of my elderly parents at the ages of 90 and 95.

It is definitely for quick study people who want all the answers immediately and don't want to spend months boning up on all the different facets of taking care of aging parents, i.e. all the medical, financial, legal and emotional issues that are pounced on you without warning.

I have given fictional names to most of the places and people that appear in this book with the exception of Mom and Dad (Liese and Leonard), my husband, Keith, my son Steve, his wife Jen, and their children Zeca and Jude, my son Adam and his wife Camilla, my brother Mick, my late sister-in-law Ellen and my niece and nephew, Colin and Nate.

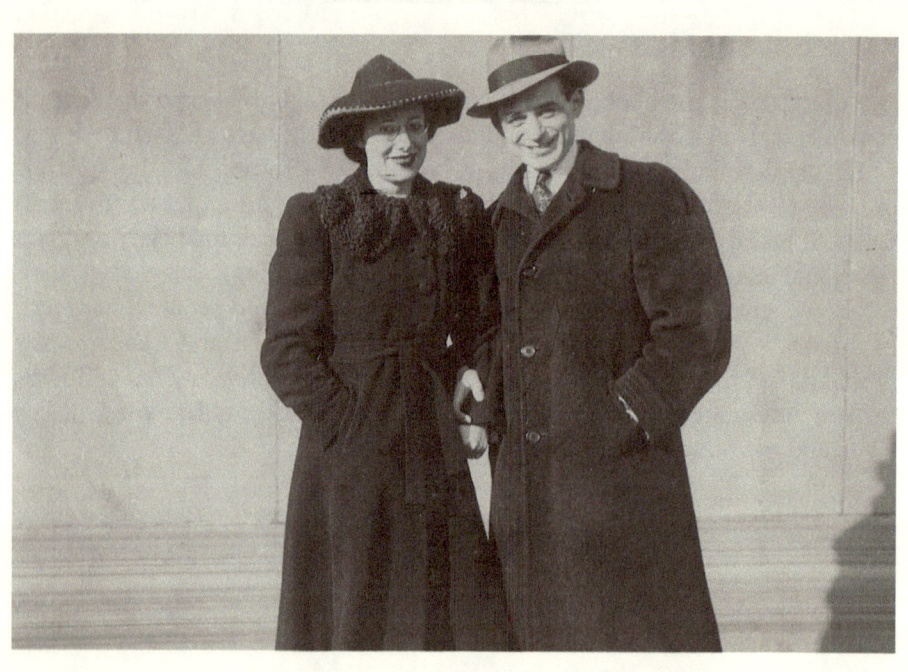

Chapter One

The Beginning

Here we are again in another crisis. Mom's in rehab. Dad is disoriented. My brother and sister-in-law are at their wit's end, and I am hundreds of miles away in Denver.

February 2011

Mom is in the Hospital

I am in Los Angeles for my cousin's 75th birthday party celebration when I get a call from my brother in Chicago that Mom has fallen and has been sent to the hospital.

"She's OK," he says.

"What happened?" I query. "Colin (my niece) was taking Mom to the bathroom and Mom fell and bumped her head. Colin couldn't get her up and so she called 911 to come and get Mom."

"I'll be there as soon as I can get home, repack, and fly out." I reply.

For the remainder of my LA trip, I am on the phone constantly with my brother, my dad, and with the doctor's office, the hospital nurses and the staff at the senior facility where Mom and Dad are living.

"If your mother stays in the hospital for three days, Medicare will pay for her to go to skilled nursing care for 100 days," says the hospital social worker. "I suggest you call her doctor and ask him to allow her to stay for the three days so she can have this service."

I hang up and immediately e-mail the doctor. This always seems to work much better than staying on the phone line and waiting or leaving a message and hoping he'll call back in some sort of timely fashion.

I get the approval and call back the social worker to notify her of the doctor's consent.

"To which nursing facility would you like to send her?"

"What are my choices?" I ask. "Doesn't Pleasant Hills have a skilled nursing unit?" Mom and Dad are living in a continuing care facility.

"They do," she replies.

"Then send her there," I decree from my hotel room in California. At the time it seemed like the best choice because then she and Dad would be in the same building and their caregivers would be able to continue to care for both of them. After all, that's why they call them continuing care residences.

March 2011

Chicago

As is my usual routine, I fly into Midway Airport rather than O'Hare because the airfare to there is cheaper. I then rent a car, and make the forty-five minute drive to the north suburbs where my parents are living. I schedule my visit from Monday to Friday to see how to assess the damages and consider future plans. I have made several appointments to visit some alternative housing facilities for Mom. Whatever I do needs to be done before I return to Denver. Our second grandchild is due any day and I need to be back home as quickly as possible.

It's a gloomy day in Chicago. I drive up I-94, stop at Whole Foods for a quick lunch, buy Mom and her caregivers African violets, one of Mom's favorite flowers, and head to Pleasant Hills. I walk through the first set of automatic doors, past the benches where several of the residents are seated and conversing, to the reception area. Though I have seen the receptionist many times before in the year and a half that Mom and Dad have lived there, she does not acknowledge my presence and only buzzes me in after I enter my name on the sign-in sheet.

I walk into the familiar foyer with its massive, calming fountain, its surrounding cushioned seats and the open view of the dining room that is dormant at the moment. Missing are the line-up of wheelchairs and residents bearing walkers that will appear at the evening meal in around an hour.

I head toward the bank of elevators around the corner. Only a few caregivers are accompanying their "charges." It's just after naptime. I get off the elevator on the sixth floor and turn down the hall to the last apartment in the nearest wing. I open the door and am greeted by my father and Condoleeza, Mom and Dad's caregiver. Condoleeza is a dream. A Filipino immigrant, she is married to an American, her second husband, with whom she has a nine year old active son. She also has three children from a previous marriage. One of her daughters, Annie, has recently arrived from the Philipines and we have hired her to take the evening shift with Mom for six days each week. Condoleeza is beautiful. Her black, thick hair is always pulled back into a tidy bun. She wears contemporary clothes in a simple style, mostly neutral turtleneck sweaters and nicely fitted jeans. She always speaks directly to you in a soft-spoken manner and though she is from another country, she seems to get the American rhythm. Dad adores her. She is always so respectful to him and makes him feel like he's the most important person in the world.

We all hug when we see each other. Dad looks a little confused. Condoleeza as always is calm and collected. She has waited to greet me before she leaves her nine to three shift. Her daughter Annie, who takes the next shift, has already gone downstairs to the skilled care unit to be with Mom. I ask Condoleeza about Mom's situation and she fills me in. Of course, she doesn't care much for how Mom is being treated in skilled care. I tell her she's my eyes and my ears, and she seems to appreciate my respect for her opinion and for the work she's doing.

Before she leaves, she turns to my dad. "Is there anything else you need, Mr. Rothman?" He pleasantly responds that he is just fine.

Dad and I then go downstairs to the basement level to see Mom. It's a long walk but Dad, at 95 years, walks jauntily and shows me the way down an endless tiled corridor. He has already learned the code that buzzes and lets us both in.

On the right, a few doors from the entrance is Mom's room. It's a double room with a curtained barrier dividing the two occupants, both of who have caregivers. Mom is sitting in a chair and she is sleeping. Her caregiver turns off her cell phone and says hello and hugs me. I am holding my African violets and trying to keep them from getting crushed.

Mom, who has primary progressive aphasia, a form of dementia that includes an inability to speak, looks at me through her foggy prism and smiles and takes my hand.

"How're you doing?" I ask knowing there will be no response.

I set down the African violet on the one set of bureaus that divides the room. The quarters are very cramped and confined. There is only one other chair next to the bed. Not an ideal situation for visiting, but no matter, Mom can't talk anyway. The television in the room is turned on, but the volume is on low.

I ask Annie how Mom is doing and she says fine.

"She sleeps a lot."

As if on cue, Mom after acknowledging my presence, dozes off. She actually seems to be in pretty good shape after her fall. She's been treated for years for her high blood pressure and high cholesterol and has been taking an increasing number of medications, upwards of twenty pills. She is on a very strong pill for her high blood pressure. This medication in particular makes her groggy and unstable. Her appetite has always been good and Annie and the staff tell me quickly that it continues to be so.

My sister-in-law and my niece, who was present when Mom fell, arrive soon after Dad and I appear. My niece apologizes for not being able to handle Mom.

"I feel terrible," my niece says.

"Don't feel that way," I say. "A lot of this is beyond our control."

Shortly after they arrive, my niece and sister-in-law exit. They already have a routine of coming and going.

Dad and I stay a bit longer.

Soon after, Dad declares, "Let's go." I accept his orders and we leave.

"She doesn't recognize me," he laments as we walk back to the elevator.

After we reach the apartment, Dad works on his current mission of sorting out his papers and belongings and deciding what he wants to give away. Last year before they moved to their new senior living quarters, he wanted to give his caregiver and her family the home where he and Mom had lived for over thirty years. He's in a giving away mood.

"Where should we go to dinner?" He asks.

"How about downstairs?" I ask.

"No. I hate this place," he bellows.

We decide to go to one of his favorite restaurants for dinner. As yet I have not seen my brother. He works during the day. I figure it's better that Dad and I touch base before we bring in the rest of the crew. At this point, Dad really only wants to have a nice night out and forget all the happenings of the past couple of weeks. He decides we'll go to his favorite restaurant. I have always enjoyed my father's company and delight in his ritual of choosing the dinner, the wine, and chatting with the restaurant owners. We don't really talk about Mom.

I return to the Hampton Inn that I have stayed at many times during the past few years as my parents' needs have become greater, but not before I stop at the Safeway to pick up a couple of bottles of wine. That, I have learned, will ease the memory of the day's happenings and put things all in perspective. I open the first and try to plan out my four days. Time is money.

The Skilled Care Routine

Each day I visit Mom and try to figure out what is going on. As far as I can see, Mom's activities are limited. She sleeps on and off throughout the day and awakes for meals. Occasionally she has a therapy session. Activities are offered in a common area, but she does not attend any of them.

During the day Condoleeza checks in on Mom from time to time, but with all her duties of tending to Dad and the apartment, she really can't spend much time with Mom. Her daughter Annie comes in at 3:00 and takes over but she rarely does anything with Mom beyond taking her to the bathroom, feeding her and getting her ready at bedtime. I try to encourage her to take Mom out of the room every once in a while. With my assistance we locate a rickety wheelchair and Annie begins to occasionally wheel Mom into the unit's main area to observe some of the activities or to look at the birds in the unit's apiary.

The skilled care unit is in charge of giving out medications. Only once do I hear that Mom's doctor has visited. Most of her monitoring and supervision takes place in the skilled care unit by nurses or nurse assistants. Through Medicare, Mom is entitled to occupational, physical and speech therapy. From what I can tell, the therapists are periodically working with Mom. It's my observation that the skilled care staff does less for Mom because they know she has caregivers watching over her.

One afternoon while I am visiting I place Mom in the rickety wheelchair and wheel her into the main area for an afternoon Karaoke session. Lo and behold I actually meet Terrance, the phantom director of skilled care and assisted living. I've been looking for him since my arrival, but he always seems to be busy. Terrance reminds me of a Latin singer. He is slim and dressed in khakis and a light blue casual shirt. He is having a great time leading the skilled care residents in the Karaoke session. Wouldn't it be lovely if he put as much effort into his real position? Terrance hands over the microphone to the other caregivers who select songs of the nineties, which are not familiar to the residents. No one sings. Not that they would anyway. Most of the songs are by current bands, not even by well-known modern vocalists like Elton John or Billy Joel. I can't keep myself from blurting out, "Do you have any Frank Sinatra or Patti Page?" Next thing I know I'm leading them all in "How Much is That Doggie in the Window" but people are at least joining in. Mom, of course, can't sing, but she smiles.

The speech therapist has paid a visit to Mom and when she meets me in the hall, she goes over the exercises she is working on with Mom. Honestly, I can't imagine her improving. I also wonder where the physical and occupational therapists are.

After realizing that the director and Thea, his subservient assistant in skilled care, are constantly unavailable, I find my lifeline with Sarah, an adorable, earnest social worker. As she addresses me, she twists her auburn hair around her finger. She looks very tired. I'm not sure whether it's because she is overworked or because she is pregnant, but she definitely shows signs of "wear and tear." Regardless, I am grateful that I have finally found a communication vessel. Sarah conscientiously pours over Mom's records and tries to make some sense of what she learns. She then schedules a conference with the skilled care staff for Thursday afternoon. I am to ask my family and our caregiver to be a part of the meeting.

Note to self:
    It's up to you to "take up the reigns." Everyone else seems to be in a holding pattern.

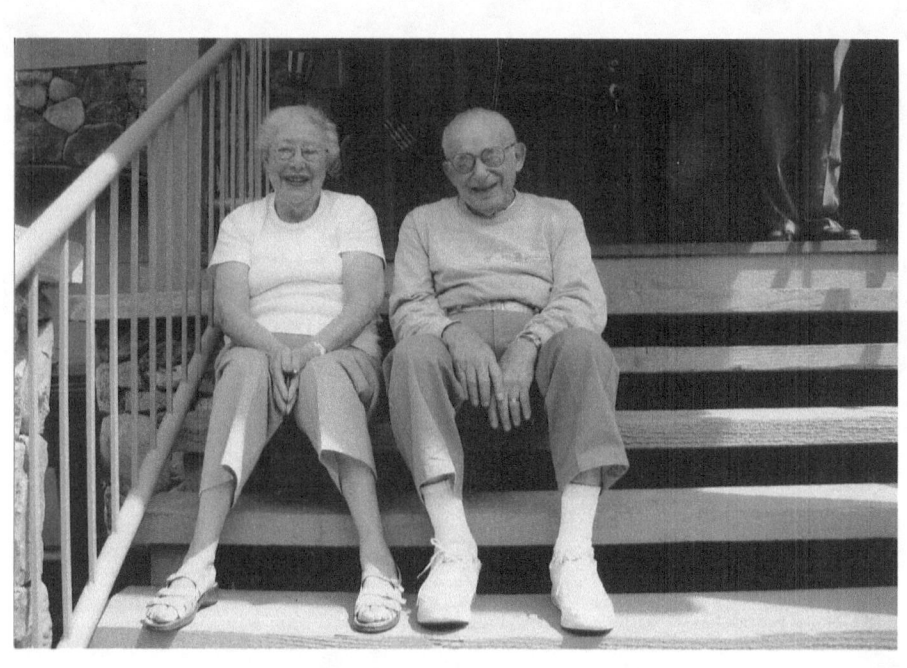

Chapter Two

How Did We Get Here?

Why can't Mom and Dad grow old together gracefully? I suppose if they've always been at loggerheads, this is just one more chapter.

The Early Golden Years

Until my mother was in her late eighties and my father was in his early nineties, my parents were totally self-reliant. They lived in a beautiful ranch home in a suburb near Chicago where they had resided for thirty years and where they entertained friends and family, and conducted a very active social life. They attended the theater and the symphony, played bridge, ate out and traveled with friends, and participated in programs at the synagogue that they had helped to start some fifty years before.

Each winter they would travel to Florida or California to be with some of their cronies and to soak up a little sunshine.

In the summer they would come and stay with us in Denver where my family had moved some thirty years prior. Throughout the rest of the year, I would make sure to see them every few months either in Chicago or at some other venue.

My brother and his family lived a few miles away from Mom and Dad. My brother would regularly check in on them to make sure they were comfortable and he and his family would usually spend their holidays together with Mom more often than not doing most of the cooking and preparation.

Mom and Dad

During and after my brother and I were growing up, Mom and Dad were always on the go.

They traveled the world. They were equally happy visiting places in the U.S. like Shipshewana, Indiana and Branson, Missouri, as they were to take cruises to Mexico or Hawaii or major global trips abroad.

Mom and Dad were attentive parents and grandparents and made sure that they attended all the milestone family events whether it was New York, San Francisco or Rio DeJaneiro. They often took us all on vacations when there were special occasions.

Mom loved to entertain and give parties. A former fashion designer, she would dress for every occasion. She had a reputation for being an inveterate shopper and for never missing a trip to a nearby outlet store. Around the house, there was always a home project going on whether it was adding on a sun room or knitting scarves and hats for everyone for the holidays or cooking and freezing her famous mushroom barley soup.

My father was equally energetic in his own style. He worked hard as a life insurance agent well into his late eighties. He rose to be president of the temple that he participated in founding. He took impeccable care of their finances and oversaw the maintenance of their home.

As a couple, my parents were charming with others, but at home they bickered continuously. They were traditional parents with my father bringing home the paychecks and my mother "ruling the roost." My mother's authoritarian German upbringing clashed with my father's egalitarian Russian socialist roots and factored into any decision that was made in the household whether it was parenting their children or deciding on how to get to the movie theater. This proved to be prescient about how they would function in their old age.

Preparing for Old Age

As they reached their late eighties and early nineties (my father was five years older than my mom), physically and medically my parents continued to be in relatively good condition. Though my mother suffered from macular degeneration and had long been on several medications to combat her high cholesterol and her high blood pressure and was prone to falling, she still managed to remain mobile. My dad's only real health issue was his prostate cancer for which he had been diagnosed more than twenty years before and for which he had received some therapy. As in the cases of many older men with the same condition, his prostate cancer was in a holding pattern and did not give him any serious difficulty.

When Mom was in her early eighties, my parents did begin to focus on where they would like to spend their final years. They retrofitted their home in anticipation of confronting old age. They moved the washer dryer and Dad's office up to the first floor and installed grab bars in the bathrooms.

Periodically they would investigate alternatives to remaining in their home. Among their friends, some had chosen to add on help as it was needed and remain in their homes while others had moved to elegant high rises that catered to seniors' needs. A few had moved into retirement communities. Mom had no interest in moving to Denver. I really believe she thought she could maintain her lifestyle forever.

It Gets Harder

There were more and more troubling incidents that kept mounting with Mom and Dad and made my brother and I realize that we were going to have to be more assertive in watching over them without cramping their independence.

First, Mom's health situation worsened. My brother took on the medical oversight for both my father and my mother. This was a gradual process but eventually he found a geriatrician to be responsible for their primary care. Ultimately the geriatrician sent Mom to a neurologist for tests and he diagnosed Mom with Primary Progressive Aphasia, a form of dementia that would eventually lead to Mom's loss of ability to speak and an increasing inability to take care of herself. Mom had a hard time accepting this. She still felt she could continue to make decisions for all of us and particularly for Dad and her.

At the onset of her diagnosis, the impact of this diagnosis did not really settle in for any of us. Eventually, though, the realization that we would once more need to reevaluate Mom and Dad's living situation began to surface. At this point Mom and Dad's active lifestyle was already changing. They canceled their season's tickets first to the symphony and soon after to the theater. They could no longer entertain as frequently or go out with friends. Though they continued to make an effort, life was definitely changing.

Mom's falls were becoming more frequent and Dad needed to help out more with the daily chores. After the house alarm went off in the middle of the night and there was a burglary on the block, I became even more concerned with how vulnerable they were to the unexpected.

One weekend Mom became dehydrated and Dad called 911 and did not notify my brother or I of the incident for several days. I knew it was time to make some changes.

Change #1: Hiring a Caregiver

After considering the retirement home facility as an option and rejecting the notion, Dad, on the recommendation of a friend, hired Condoleeza. Several years prior, Condoleeza had immigrated from the Philipines where she had been a caregiver. After she had taken classes to become certified in the States, she worked for an agency. Her children had remained in the Philipines. She hoped to bring them to America at some point in the future. In the meantime she remarried an American and had a child who was now nine-years and who was cared for by Condoleeza's sister. At this point Condoleeza preferred to work independently rather than with an agency. Amazingly, she could adapt to whatever my parents' needs might be. At the onset she worked five hours a day, five days a week. Her job was to clean, do the laundry, prepare the meals, run errands, help administer Mom's medications, and take Mom to her numerous doctor and dental appointments. Mom and Dad remained by themselves at night.

At first Condoleeza was the perfect solution to our problems. But as the months went by and Mom's condition worsened, life again took a downturn. Mom was becoming more and more aggressive and difficult, and Dad was becoming more and more depressed. They both complained to me each day when I talked to them on the phone. I spent the remainder of my day worrying about them and trying to find things for them to do to fill in the new voids in their lives. Nothing worked. The situation was becoming increasingly difficult.

Dad is Hospitalized

About a year and a half after Mom and Dad hired Condoleeza, Dad got an infection and was rushed to the hospital where he was placed in intensive care and not given much chance of surviving. My sister-in-law stayed with Mom and my brother took control at the hospital until I arrived and then I stayed for two weeks while Dad miraculously recovered. During his recuperation, we hired full time caregivers to supplement the services of their regular caregiver.

Change #2: Moving to a Senior Facility

Once again, I knew we had to do something. In between nursing Dad back to health and coping with Mom, I had just had it with all the bickering from all fronts, from my father, my mother, from Condoleeza and from my exhausted brother and sister-in-law. I decided Mom and Dad could no longer make their living decisions alone and I was going to have to involve myself more actively in trying to adjust to what was coming. Clearly in my mind, they were both going to continue to deteriorate in one way or another. My brother was still working and could not help out that much. Though my niece and nephew were living nearby both of them were working, and my sister-in-law, who had recently stopped working, had health problems of her own. I was hundreds of miles away and thus unable to fill in when necessary or to supervise Mom and Dad's situation effectively. I wanted everyone to have to worry less about getting through the day, and I wanted my brother and I to have assistance in providing comfort to them. I also thought that if Mom and Dad were in a controlled social environment that they would be happier and that they would have more to distract them from their maladies.

One morning during my two week vigil watching over Dad, I decided to take another look at Pleasant Hills, the same senior living facility they had considered after Mom had been sent to the hospital for dehydration. I was ushered around the facility by Haley who had worked with Mom and Dad a few years before when Mom thought an available apartment was too close to the elevator. Haley was the consummate saleswoman. She wore a simple black pant suit with a crisp blue cotton shirt. Her silky blonde hair was pulled back at the nape of her neck. She chatted breezily with me about Mom and Dad. "Oh yes," she crooned. "I remember your Mom and Dad. They were so adorable." She showed me a beautiful corner apartment on the top floor that looked out over the Chicago skyline. I gave her a check to hold the space and then I brought my parents back in the afternoon. Haley was there to welcome them once more and to triumphantly show them to the corner apartment. At the end of the day, my father signed the papers and gave a deposit. Even Mom nodded her approval when she saw the place.

In a month and a half, we moved Mom and Dad into their new home, put their house up for sale and brought along Condoleeza to help out with the same five hours a day, five days a week schedule.

I placed Mom and Dad each in separate bedrooms in the two bedroom apartment. This was a bit traumatic especially for Mom. We set up their furniture and art in pretty much the same configuration they had had in their old home. I thought it looked quite nice.

Condoleeza continued to serve them lunch and to do the laundry and take Mom to her doctors' appointments. She would leave at three in the afternoon and then Mom and Dad would go down to the dining hall for dinner and retire to their apartment for the night. As a means of checking in on the residents, the building required that everyone secure their doors each night and unlock them each morning. A monitoring system made sure this was done appropriately.

I felt relieved that I no longer had to worry about their safety when they were not being watched over by the caregiver and that they had a regular dinner to go to each night.

Life at Pleasant Hills

The new situation worked well for a while. Dad continued to go about his usual business. He had taken along his beloved Buick and had paid extra for a garage space. On the weekends my brother continued his normal visits on Saturday mornings and would pick them both up on Sunday nights at first to go out to eat and when Mom could no longer go out, to take them over to his house for Sunday night dinner. My dad's best friend continued to be Condoleeza.

Dad tolerated his new surroundings but he wasn't very happy. He didn't like the people. They were all too old and he didn't like anything else about the place. To be honest, the move had been a trade-off. Living in a controlled environment was safer and more predictable but there was something missing. We knew of several other people who lived at Pleasant Hills and were very happy there, but Dad's temperament was not as easy going. I think Mom enjoyed the socialization aspect more than Dad who liked his privacy, his projects and his own choice of company.

More Problems and More Caregiving

Unfortunately soon after they moved, Mom's condition, as predicted, worsened even moreso, and she needed more care. She began to have difficulty dressing herself and performing her daily functions. Dad would tell me that she made herself breakfast at three in the morning. Oftentimes when I would visit, she would be standing at the open door of her apartment aimlessly gazing out into the hallway. I was grateful that she did not wander into the hall, but I also worried that crossing over that line might be her next move.

Condoleeza would report that Mom was becoming more and more disoriented and often was physically aggressive.

We decided to hire more caregivers and eventually arrived at a situation where six days a week, both day and night, Condoleeza and Annie, her daughter, split the duties, and on Sundays my niece came in and took over.

The round the clock caregiving was helpful but Mom was becoming more and more difficult to handle, and Dad was helplessly watching all of this take place while they both remained in the same apartment.

I Need Help!

At this point I decided to contact Senior Works, a Chicago company that I had initially been introduced to at the time Mom and Dad moved to Pleasant Hills. Owned by Heather, the same woman who operated the moving company that specialized in helping seniors to move, Heather had been working in the senior care field for many years. In my mind she skillfully operated her for profit company that consulted the elderly and their caregivers, guided them on how to handle the difficult problems that arise during the aging process and then steered them to helpful services that were screened and approved of by her. The businesses paid a fee for belonging to the network. Until we hired a service, the assistance was free.

At Christmastime before Mom's fall, my husband and I had met at a nearby Starbucks with Helen, one of Senior Works' social workers, to discuss our current dilemma. Professional in manner with a quiet sense of gravitas, Helen peered out over wireless glasses that framed her lightly lined face and listened empathetically to our concerns about Dad's depression, the continuing deterioration of Mom's status including accelerating attacks of violence, and our worry about the increasing costs of caregivers.

I reviewed the circumstances that had led to Mom and Dad's move from their comfortable family home into their current senior facility a year and a half prior.

Helen listened carefully but was non-committal.

"It is very common for elderly couples to have different health issues and to be at different stages," she said. "Depending on the couples' personalities, the solution should be solved in different ways." Though she did point out a few alternatives on how to proceed, mostly it was a back and forth about what were the circumstances. She did suggest visiting a facility for Dad that she thought might be a better "fit." From our discussion with her, I started to think that maybe it might be better for Mom and Dad to live near each other but in separate facilities.

Encouraged by our meeting with Helen, my husband and I quickly followed up on her suggestion and went to visit the facility she had recommended for Dad. We instantly fell in love with the place and tried to encourage Dad to visit the facility. He would have nothing to do with the suggestion and ultimately canceled an appointment we made for him to visit the place.

Perhaps Helen's suggestion to live in separate quarters was too "clinical." I myself was torn about changing Mom and Dad's living arrangements again. Mom and Dad's closest friends who had had differences in their aging issues all seemed to be able to handle disparities and stay together. But Dad was impatient and Mom was beginning to be impossible to handle. They had always had their differences, and their difficulty in getting along was becoming more and more heightened.

I decided to keep things as they were. We had made our decision and we needed to live with it.

Then Mom fell and wound up in skilled care and we were forced to regroup.

Note to self: Am I overthinking the situation? Why don't I just "go with the flow" and wait for the next disaster to occur and address the situation when it comes up?

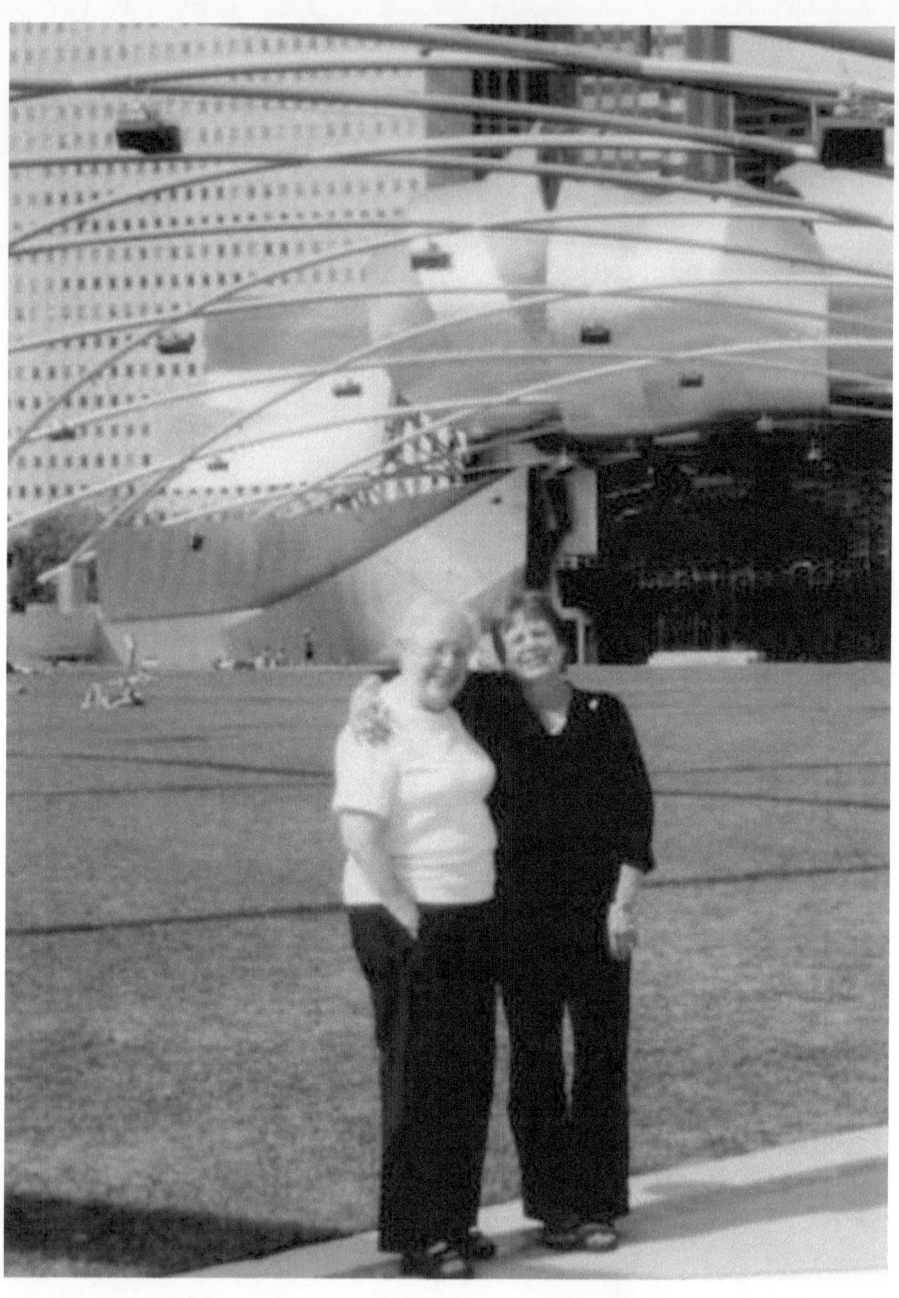

Chapter Three

Chicago

To change their living situations or not to change their living situations? That is the question.

We Go Searching—Day One

After my return from LA and before leaving for Chicago, I had once more contacted Heather at Senior Works, the agency my husband and I had visited at Christmas. She referred me back to Helen, the social worker we had met at Starbucks, and I then called her and asked her for recommendations on possible alternative living options to consider for Mom and that I could investigate when I came to Chicago to visit Mom. She had given me a list and I had followed up and made appointments to visit most of the establishments she suggested.

Elegant Assisted Living

On the morning after the first day I arrive, I go to a lovely facility in a suburb nearby where Mom and Dad are living. I meet Marilyn, the exquisitely dressed director of the facility with whom I have made the appointment. She has advanced degrees in social work and gerontology and she knows her stuff. The facility is privately owned and has a sister independent living facility located in another nearby community. It turns out that I am at the sister facility to the independent facility we visited for

Dad at Christmastime and which he rejected. A van regularly transports the independent residents from the other facility back and forth to visit their loved ones in the assisted living facility.

We chat for quite a while about Dad and Mom's situation and she takes me around to see the grounds. In contrast to Pleasant Hills, the atmosphere is very subdued and low key. I agree to bring Dad back the next day to get his "take".

Apartments for Dad?

After my visit to the first assisted living facility, I drive around and look at some of the apartments for Dad in the nearby area where some of Mom and Dad's friends live. Nothing appeals. I worry about letting Dad live on his own with no grocery stores, no shopping area and no easily accessible avenues for socialization. He would have to drive everywhere or take a cab, something I could never see him doing.

We Go Searching—Day Two

The next day Dad and I and my sister-in-law go to one of the other places recommended for Mom by Senior Works. It is a religious affiliated facility (we are Jewish). Instantly I can tell that my mother would not be happy here. The place smells of Lysol and there is no carpeting on the floor. Women in their wheelchairs are gathered in clusters gossiping in English and sometimes Yiddish. My mother, a German Jew, even with dementia would never approve. Not only that, but I can hear cries for help coming from some of the rooms.

Then we move on to the facility that I had visited the day before where we are served coffee and cookies in the lobby (very civilized!) before Marilyn, the director, comes out to meet with us. She is so deferential to Dad and treats him with great respect.

"Would you like a wheelchair while I'm showing you around?" She inquires.

Dad, of course, says no and displays his jauntiest walk. She shows us a few independent units on the first floor where Dad could stay if he preferred rather than commuting from their other independent living facility. She introduces us to Mrs. Peters who had moved to the first floor from the sister independent living facility several years ago when her husband who has since passed away became a resident. She is now over one hundred years old and continues to remain in her apartment. "I just needed a little something more," she explains as she proudly shows us around her meticulous apartment that is decorated in floral patterns. She is one feisty lady.

Dad takes it all in. To be honest, I can't imagine Dad assessing his own needs!

After lunch, we return to Pleasant Hills. Dad naps while Haley, the blonde, attractive saleswoman who originally placed Mom and Dad at Pleasant Hills and is currently five months pregnant, takes me on a tour of the third choice on the social worker's list, Pleasant Hills' smaller independent living facilities for Dad and the assisted living area for Mom. Haley characteristically displays her hyperbolic enthusiasm.

"I love this studio," she beams. "We have great studios." This, after reminding me of Pleasant Hills "five star rating." (With whom, I wonder?)

"No bad views," she continues as she shows me another available studio.

After we tour the independent facilities, we move on to the assisted living quarters where Mom would live if she were to remain at Pleasant Hills. I can just imagine her walking down the long corridors and looking for the dining area. I knew Mom would still need a caregiver, which would make the cost accelerate substantially. It also bothered me that the director of the assisted living quarters was Terrance, the phantom director of the skilled care unit where Mom was currently housed.

My Brother Announces That He is Leaving Chicago

In the middle of my stay in Chicago, my brother informs me that he and his family have decided to move to Albuquerque next June when he retires and that he will no longer be able to be the daily point man if Mom and Dad have any emergencies.

With no one to take care of Mom and Dad on a daily basis, we will have to rely on caregivers and the senior housing facility where they live. Though this scenario will not take place for a little over a year, it does mean that whatever decision we make about Mom and Dad will have to include this additional "glitch" and will force us to find more local supervision once my brother is no longer in Chicago.

My regular caregiving routine had been to travel every three months to make sure things were in place and then to make special trips for emergencies. In between trips I had been coordinating with Mom and Dad and the caregiver over the phone. I am very uncomfortable with the idea of my brother not being there to back me up if there is an emergency. After considering the idea of temporarily returning to Chicago to take care of them, I decide that for now we will just have to try to find a comfortable situation that will work and deal with the supervision problem later.

Where We Leave It

On my last night in Chicago, I head back to the Hampton Inn, drink wine, try to sleep and wake up intermittently. At one point, I just get up and try to work on possible future scenarios for Mom and Dad. This has been a very difficult stay.

Before I leave on Thursday, I pack up for my return trip to Denver, put my suitcase in the car, and head over to say good by to Mom and attend the conference that was set up in skilled care with the help of Sarah, the social worker and which is intended to address Mom's needs and help us come up with a plan for the future.

Not much happens at the conference. Terrance, the director, is a no show and everyone else just goes through the motions. Thea, the assistant director drones on and on about Mom's eating and sleeping habits. "Liese seems to have a healthy appetite although she tends to choke." We all know this already. Condoleeza, our devoted caregiver, patiently listens as do the rest of us including, Dad, my brother, my sister-in-law and myself. We all decide to do our best, whatever that means.

I say good-by to Mom and everyone else and we agree to keep working on coming up with some sort of solution to our current situation and to just keep things going for the time being.

I decide to contact Mom's doctor to see what he thinks would be the best situation just from a medical point of view. I am already back in Denver when the doctor replies that he thinks because of Mom's tendency to fall she would need twenty-four hour supervision.

I also decide to call the last name on the list of possibilities that I had not been able to reach initially. From Denver I get in touch with the director of the facility and she turns out to be the best interview and to be the best candidate for accommodating Mom's needs. She immediately grasps the details about Mom's circumstances and easily convinces me that her home would work for Mom. The facility is a small, privately owned operation and is well located. I call my sister-in-law and ask her to go over and look at the place. She promises to do so soon. I feel that cost-wise and care-wise, this place might be the answer for Mom. My sister-in-law never makes it over there before Plan B is put into effect.

Note to self: Take some time out and mull all this over. You need some distance.

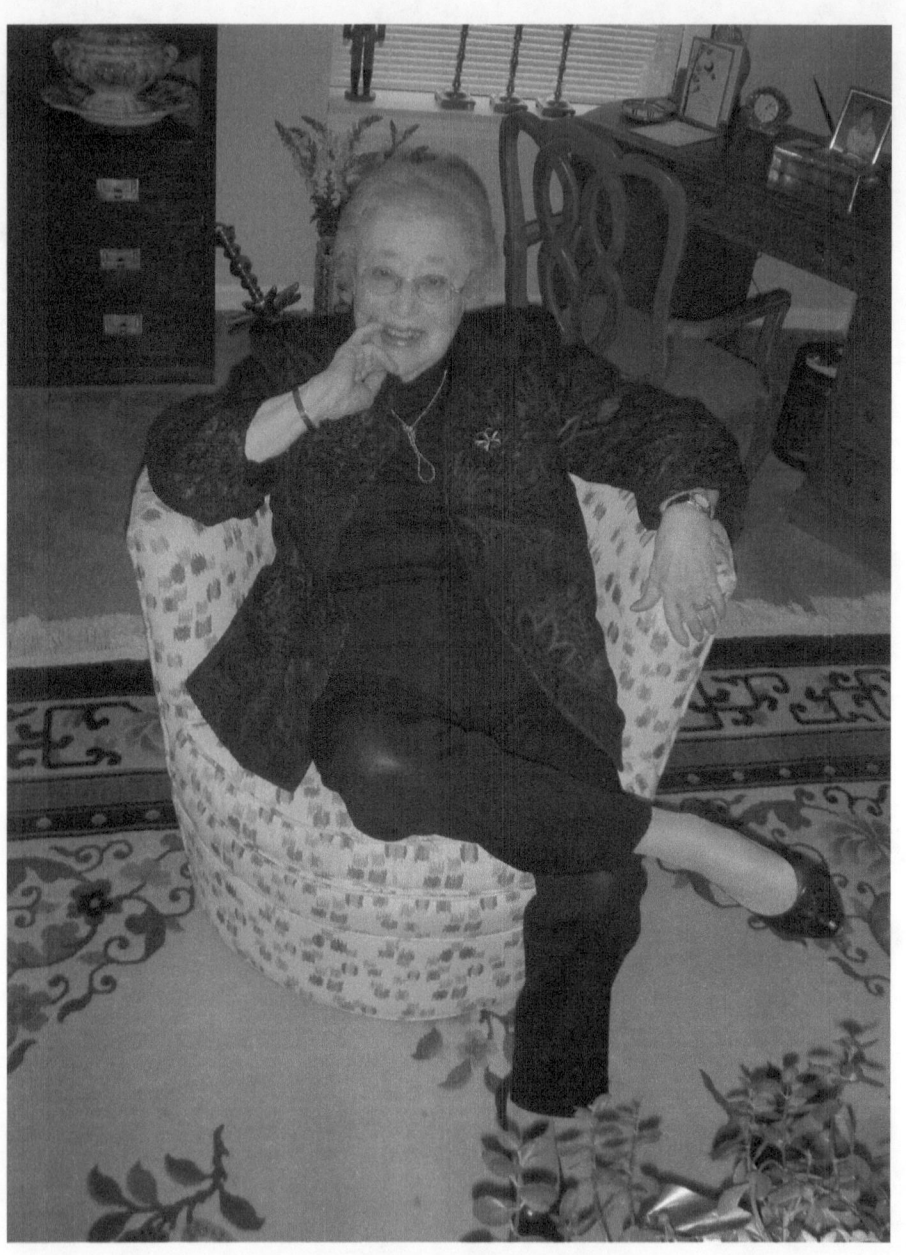

Chapter Four

Taking Stock

So my brother is moving to Albuquerque when he retires. Who'd have thunk it? It's back to the drawing table.

The Current Situation

After being in Chicago for five days with my parents, my brother and sister-in-law and my niece and nephew, and, after getting some information from the staff at the skilled care unit, I am now reviewing everyone's concerns, needs and feelings and trying to come up with a solution.

I know that Medicare will pay for Mom to remain in skilled care for a limited time as long as she keeps improving and that after her time is up, she will either have to return to her residence at Pleasant Hills or we will have to find some place else for her to live.

I need to decide as quickly as possible where Mom and Dad should reside in the future. Together? Apart? At Pleasant Hills? At what cost?

I have discussed the matter with my father who is trying to maintain some sort of schedule and visit Mom daily. Understandably, he is quite disoriented and not really of much help.

My brother and sister-in-law are just happy to get through each day and at this point weary from the need to react to the continuing demise of both parents. The announcement that they will be moving to New Mexico has further complicated the situation.

Sarah, the social worker at the skilled nursing facility has reported to me that Mom is getting a bit of speech therapy and other than that, she is entirely in a holding pattern. That means she is eating, sleeping, and taking a lot of pills and that's it.

Naturally Condoleeza would like to continue taking care of Mom and Dad.

Though Condoleeza is a wonderful caregiver, and Dad adores her, she is not trained to make medical decisions or to analyze Mom's current living situation. Of course she has opinions that I welcome and I am very happy that she and her daughter are continuing to take such good care of Mom during this crisis period.

Priorities

Based on my discussions with all involved and with Helen, the social worker from Senior Works, I create a list of priorities to help me determine how to proceed.

The issues that I believe need to be addressed include 1) Mom and Dad's medical and emotional states, 2) Money, 3) Mom's security, 4) Supervision for both of them, 5) The easiest solution for my brother and myself, and 6) Practically speaking how quickly we can expedite a solution.

Medical and Emotional Needs

Mom's situation is the most dire. She is basically living like a vegetable. She is inert, incontinent and barely aware of her surroundings. She can no longer speak except in monosyllables and she cannot govern her daily life. Her medications subdue her aggressive tendencies but they also keep her so sedated that she sleeps constantly.

Dad continues to remain capable of taking care of himself, but he is unhappy with his current living situation. His only solace comes from his Friday afternoon bridge game and from his one on one chats with Condoleeza. He often tells me he wants to "get out of this place" (referring to Pleasant Hills) and get his own apartment or move in with a lady friend of his and Mom's. He has even gone so far as to call a realtor friend to inquire about locating an apartment where he can live independently. This is not the first time he has considered this option. In the past he thought maybe he and my niece and nephew could all rent an apartment together. I can only foresee trouble if he decides to live independently. When these moments occur I pose questions to him regarding such issues as who would help him take care of the house, who would make his meals, and what kind of safety net would he have if he had an emergency? Sometimes this uncertainty will temporarily quiet down his desire to pursue any of these options. Dad's situation is less of a concern to me than Mom's. We need to resolve her situation first, and then we can move on to Dad.

Do We Have Enough Money?

So far we had been very fortunate that Dad, a retired life insurance salesman has done a good job of managing his and Mom's finances. Dad's income consists of his and Mom's Social Security payments, an annuity, and interest from their investments. Though he has not yet had to draw down their principal even with the additional cost of the caregivers, if we decide to change Mom and Dad's living situations, the expenses will more than likely increase and at that time we will have to start digging into their principal.

After doing the calculations for the various costs of care, I decide that regardless of which way we go and if I am careful at allocating the expenses, we probably have enough money to cover the next five to seven years before the money runs out.

Security, Supervision, Caregiving

Whatever choices I make, the bottom line is that they both need to be in situations where they are not in any form of danger, where someone is checking in on them regularly, and where, if an emergency arises, someone will be able to navigate the situation and get them to the proper facility. Mom must have somebody take care of all of these concerns, and Dad, although very alert, will need help in making any kind of decisions regarding these issues.

As for caregiving, both my brother and I are fortunate in the sense that we can afford to pay for others to watch over our parents, but as in any situation where employees are hired, rarely is anyone as caring or concerned as the one who is in charge of the caregiving, i.e. the supervising family member.

Bringing About Change

For some reason, I always think that any decision made can be managed. It may not be easy, but it can be done. This should be the very least of my concerns.

The Choices

I boil down the options based on the list of priorities I have determined to be most important.

The first alternative to consider is for Mom to return to their two-bedroom apartment and continue with the 24/7 caregiving. The advantage to this would be that she would be in familiar territory. The disadvantage would be that life would continue to be very unpleasant for everyone involved and that it would be just a matter of time before she would fall again and be sent to the ER.

The second alternative would be for Mom to remain at the same facility as Dad but to move into the assisted living section rather than remain in the independent living quarters where they are currently living. She would be given three meals a day and she would be aided with dressing and bathing and getting ready for bed at night and she would have the option of participating in activities designed for those people who are also in the assisted living unit. In that scenario, Dad would then just move to a studio or one-bedroom in the same facility. The advantage of that choice would be that they would not have to be going to a strange new place again, and that they would be near one another in the same building. The disadvantage to that choice would be that Mom would not have 24/7 supervision unless we continued to employ our caregivers to watch over Mom. The assisted living unit at Pleasant Hills is not a separate unit just for people with dementia, a concept that is unfamiliar to me at the time. If left on her own, Mom would still be free to move about as she pleased. Moving Mom to assisted living with additional caregiving would be a very costly option.

Another possibility would be for Mom to continue to live in the senior living facility's very small skilled care unit, which is secure, but no private apartment is currently available. This would mean she would just continue to stay in her current double occupancy room. I do not consider moving Mom into a nursing home, which, though very confining, might have been another alternative and something in retrospect I should have investigated. The Senior Works' social worker does not suggest this either.

A fourth alternative would be to move Mom to some place that could better handle her needs. In that scenario, we would decide on where Dad would live based on what we found for Mom. That would mean shuttling back and forth between Mom and Dad's living quarters and it would also mean that they were no longer together in the same place.

Note to self: Get over making the perfect decision. There is none.

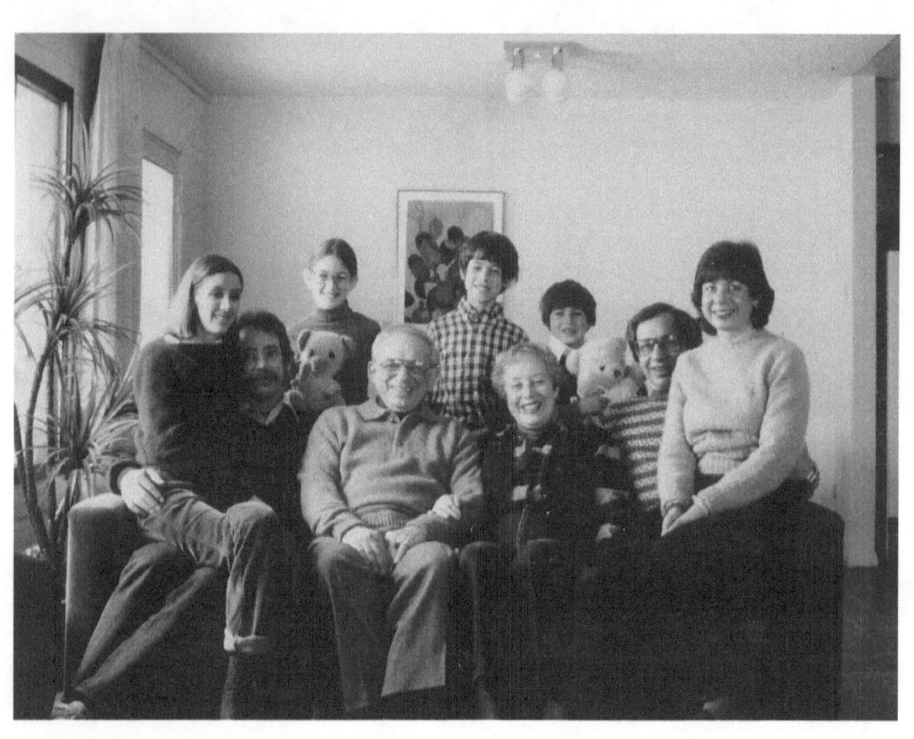

Chapter Five

Plan B: How About Denver?

After all that searching in Chicago, would you believe I'm considering moving them to Denver?

Late March 2011

I am back in Denver for the birth of our second grandson. Nothing is better than that!

Shortly after I return, I go to get my regular haircut and lament to my hairdresser about my parents' situation. My hairdresser is a thirty something single girl with parents in Toronto.

She says to me, "I wish my parents would move to Denver so I could take care of them. Why don't you bring your parents to Denver?"

I have never thought about this as a possibility. My mom had indoctrinated into me many years ago before she lost her ability to talk that she didn't want to live in Denver. Now that circumstances have changed, I think I might need to override her. I decide to run across the idea to my husband first. This would be a huge commitment on our part and he would be deeply involved in such a choice. He seemed fine with it.

Then I run it by my brother before I approach Dad with the idea. My brother has no problem buying in to the idea either. After all, he is leaving Chicago anyway and Denver will actually be a lot closer to his new Albuquerque residence.

"Dad," I say over the phone. "I have an idea that I want to run by you. What do you think of coming out to Denver?"

He laughs his deep gruff laugh. "Where would Mom go?" He then asks.

"With you. She'd come out here too." (I think to myself, "She may not be happy, but she has no choice.") He seems to like the idea immediately.

Then I follow up.

"I'm going to write down the pros and cons and e-mail them to you," I say. (Dad is still using his computer at this point.)

I draw up a list of the pros and cons and the three of us, my dad, my brother and I go over the list carefully:

PROS AND CONS FOR NEW LIVING ARRANGEMENTS:

OPTION A—Mom and Dad stay in Chicago

Pros:
1) Would be the least jarring as far as change is concerned.
2) My brother and his wife would be on hand to make dinners on Sunday for the time being and to take Mom to some of her doctor and dentist appointments.
3) Mom and Dad would still be able to get together with old friends.

Cons:
1) My brother and his wife plan to move in less than two years and when they do, no one will be around to offer constant supervision.
2) At that point the visitation by both children and their families would occur at the minimum of every few months.
3) All other problems would have to be taken care of by phone.

OPTION B—Mom and Dad move to Colorado

Pros:
1) Mimi would be around to monitor the situation and to handle any needed changes as they would occur.
2) Mom and Dad could see their grandchildren and their great grandchildren.
3) We would not have to worry about Mom and Dad being left alone in Chicago in two years without support.

Cons:
1) The initial move would be somewhat jarring and costly.
2) Mom and Dad would each have to adjust, Dad to finding a new routine in independent living, Mom to getting comfortable in a new environment.

OPTION C—Mom stays in Chicago and Dad Moves to Colorado

Pros:
1) Mom is more comfortable being in Chicago and wouldn't be as happy in Colorado.
2) Dad could try a new life since he is not that pleased living at Pleasant Hills.
3) He would enjoy being with our Denver family and his extended family.
4) My husband and I would enjoy having him here and make sure that he had things to do.

Cons:
1) I think it would be hard on both Mom and Dad to be separated.
2) Dad could turn out not to like living in Colorado any better than he does living in Chicago.
3) Even if Dad were to move, everything would be new and he would have to get used to a lot of things.

The cost factor turned out to be pretty much of a wash. Ironically it was much more expensive for them to live in Chicago, but moving costs would be greater and would add on expenses at the onset.

I worry much more about the costs than anyone else does.

My dad buys into the idea of moving to Denver immediately. My brother, as you can well imagine, likes the idea too!

Then it is time to begin the search for where my parents will live all over again, but this time it is in Denver! My head is spinning. What kind of facility can we find for them? How will we get them here? How can we pack them up? How will we tell Mom? How soon can we make this happen? I decide to take one piece of the puzzle at a time.

Note to self: I am so happy with our decision. I'm even happier that we went through the process and let everyone weigh in with their opinions. I think I can handle the details. Why am I not more worried?

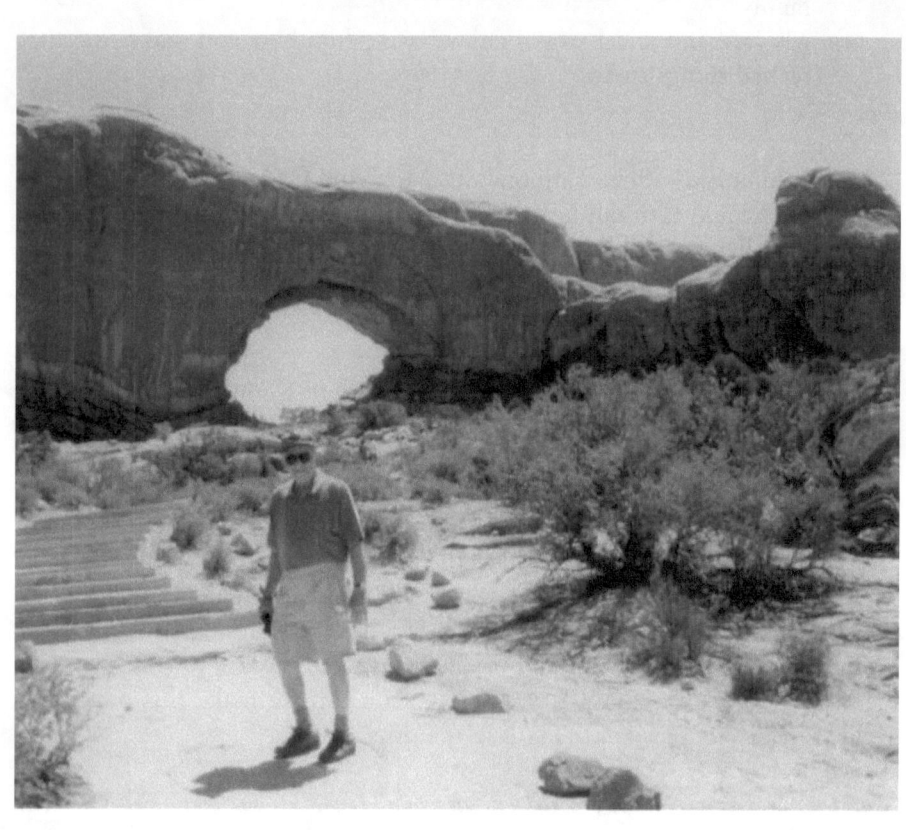

Chapter Six

Search II: Denver

Guess what? I'm repeating the search for places for them to live but this time it's in Denver. I have one week to decide. Oh well, at least I know the drill. It's an unconventional choice, but it seems right for our circumstances.

April 2011

Now that I have decided that the folks will move to Denver, I again begin a search to find a place for them to live and attempt to see how quickly I can make this happen. I decide to worry about the latter part after I find them a place to live.

From my Chicago search I had worked out in my mind what kind of living situation would be best for each. I felt Mom would need to be in some sort of dementia unit and Dad would have to live in independent living in a senior facility. In my new assertive manner, I ruled out the thought of him having his own apartment.

Another Senior Living Agency

Having been so pleased with Senior Works, the Chicago resource senior service agency, I again take to the internet to look around for a similar service in Denver. There are all kinds of websites, all more than willing to help you. It takes a little time to find the one I choose, a national franchise that provides options for you and is supported by the service providers who are screened by the agency and who pay a fee to be recommended by the agency. I'm working with a woman named Susan. She is communicative and responsive.

First she asks me what my needs are which I share with her: I need some place close; I need some place soon; I prefer some place where both parents can be housed; I need some place for Mom that can deal with her dementia. Along with her suggestions I also make up a list of recommendations from people I know in my community who are taking care of elderly parents or who have done so in the past.

I share this information with Susan and then, based on her and my recommendations, she makes up a list of places for me to visit. Then she schedules the appointments. One week after my return from Chicago, I repeat the same type of rounds except this time the tours are in Denver!!!

Choice One: Small Assisted Living

First, I visit two different venues just for Mom that exclusively accept dementia patients. One is a house in a residential neighborhood where about seven to ten residents live in a cozy little "nest." It's a little bit too "down home" and a little bit too intimate for my taste. It reminds me of pre-school. Lots of dolls and stuffed animals. The man who owns the facility operates several others just like it around the same area fairly close to where we live. I think he's a former medical professional who decided to start a string of these homes as a business.

The second place I go to for Mom is in the suburbs but again not too far away. This is a newer building that kind of resembles a summer resort. It has the usual caregivers and the usual facilities, a room for each resident, a kitchen, which serves them all meals, and general areas to congregate in. One man is walking around the place with no trousers, a bit much for me. The atmosphere is very low key, but it just doesn't feel right. Something's missing, but I'm not sure what. I think the atmosphere is just not upbeat.

Neither of these facilities does much for me. I'm not sure why. They just don't feel right.

Choice Two: A Corporate Facility

Then I go to visit a facility owned by a large national company that would be able to accommodate both Mom and Dad. It's about a twenty to thirty minute drive away. The dementia unit is extremely impressive. Both the marketing director and the executive director who are trained in gerontology usher me through a beautiful facility that seems totally under control and very comfortably outfitted. The independent living arm of the facility seems a little bit stuffy to me, but it has all the amenities, i.e. the coffee bar/grocery, the long list of activities, a beautifully furnished dining room that would be good for Dad. This is the most expensive facility I visit.

More Choices

In the next few days, I visit two places for Dad. The first is a joint independent living/assisted living facility that is religiously funded. It is a not for profit organization. Whether or not you are on Medicaid, you can live in this facility. Only blocks from our house, the complex had been in existence for many years. It has a very large common area with a very nice outdoor space. The residents seem quite independent and comfortable. The ambience, though it has recently been improved, seems a bit spare to me.

I consider it a possibility.

The next place I visit had been the past residence for my daughter-in-law's now deceased grandfather who lived there only a short time when he came to Denver before he became ill and passed away.

Here I lunch with Sally, the marketing assistant, a very personable young woman, who explains to me that Dad could live in this facility and a bus could take him to see Mom in a sister facility not too far away that serves residents with dementia. It's easy to connect with Sally. She seems to know a lot of the same people that I know, a point that works in her favor.

The facility has two components: assisted living and independent living. The atmosphere is energetic. People mull around the coffee bar, inquire at the front desk about excursions to the grocery store and cultural events. The dining room is bright and the residents upbeat. This would be a perfect place for Dad, but the drawback is that they cannot accommodate Mom's needs.

The One

Lastly, my husband accompanies me to the one remaining facility on the short list. (There were others to consider, but only if the top choices weren't acceptable.) Here we are met by Midge, a stunning woman who is filling in for the regular marketing manager and visiting from corporate headquarters in Boston. Her auburn hair is fashionably styled and she wears a knit suit that looks like a St. John's. She chatters personably about how much she's enjoying visiting Denver. My husband and I love that cosmopolitan touch! The facility she shows us is only five minutes away from us. It is a high rise building with eighteen floors. The second floor houses the dementia unit, assisted living is on the second and third floors and the remaining other residents (five hundred total) live in a variety of independent housing apartments (the second to the top floor is an expansive penthouse and the top floor is an airy party room with a view of the city). On the bottom floor there's a swimming pool, a card and meeting room and a beauty salon and barbershop. On the main floor there are all kinds of traditionally furnished rooms in which to gather, a beautifully appointed dining room and, most important to my husband, (and really to me too) a bar!!!!!

Everyone here seems to be having a great time. Yes, there are a lot of people walking around with walkers or in wheelchairs. Yes, caregivers accompany many. It just doesn't seem to matter. There are a lot of nicely dressed, smiling people mulling around the place.

We take the final choice immediately. There are a number of reasons for this. Obviously it's a beautiful facility that has been in existence for over twenty years and has a very upbeat atmosphere. Secondly, it is only five minutes from our home. Most importantly, it can house both Mom and Dad. They will be in different units but they can see each other any time.

I'm not sure whether I know at the time that the facility is owned by one of the largest senior living companies in the country. I do recall being aware that it was a for profit organization and that it did not take Medicaid. I figured that we would make another move if the money ran out. I think I considered the fact that the facility was a money making corporation to be a plus. Since they had been in business for many years, I thought they would be the most knowledgeable about the ins and outs of caring for the elderly, could anticipate more readily the needs of its residents, and would be familiar with how to handle any crisis that might arise. The fact that they seemed to have people waiting to get into the facility reinforced my feeling that this was the right place for Mom and Dad. I don't think I addressed many of the nuances or services or policies at the time. That might have been a good idea and saved me some aggravation later. (See chapter on "Reflections.") I doubt it would have made any difference in my choice, but it might have made a difference in my preparation. I really thought this was the right place and certainly my husband did.

I think the agency we used did a good job. If I had not been under such a time crunch, I probably could have been more thorough in my investigation, but considering the deadlines we were dealing with, even when I look back, I think I made the right choice.

Note to self: I'm comfortable going with my gut. Am I working too fast? You've already made a commitment. Just keep going.

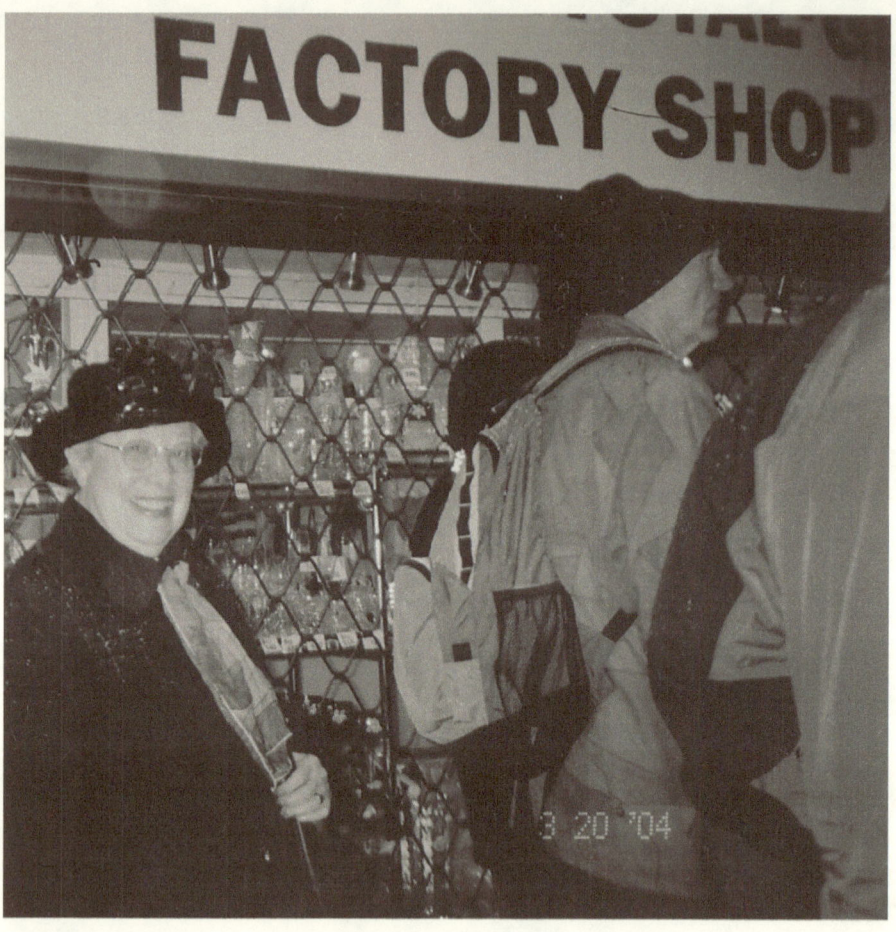

Chapter Seven

Moving

The goal is to get them to the mile high city in six weeks. The to do list is a mile high too. I'm going to have to be organized and creative.

April to May 2011

Where to Begin

Now it's time to figure out the logistics of how to condense Mom and Dad's belongings and pack them up, but I can't do this until I have filled out mounds of paper work required to get them to Denver. There is a bulging packet from their new living facility, and another packet from the facility they will be leaving. There are medical reports, living wills and do not resuscitate forms, personal history forms and many consent forms. The paper work is all done from Denver. I ask my brother and sister-in-law to secure Mom and Dad's complete medical records in Chicago. Of course, that doesn't quite get done until I spend several more hours on this project alone once I get to Chicago to pick up my parents.

For their new residence, I read the contracts and tremble with fear as I write out the check for the $3,000 entrance fee as well as for the first month's rents for each of them. I am very happy that I have had experience as a business owner in my prior life and that my attorney husband is there for me if I have any reservations at all. I am grateful that the new senior facility will waive the second entrance fee for Dad. I don't think the facility very often sees two parents at my parents' age entering their system.

For each parent I figure out what furniture to take based on the layouts of each of their units. When Mom and Dad had moved into their current living quarters, the director Selma spent a whole day cutting up tiny pieces of paper to scale and moved them around the apartment blueprint to try to arrange each room in the most attractive configuration. This time it's a bit more of an eyeball strategy. Maybe the past laborious efforts help me figure out how to do this in a quicker, more efficient manner.

I give notification to their current facility and work with their staff to sever their lease. This proves to be a very uncomfortable situation. All of those lovely people who have been so kind and friendly to us during Mom and Dad's stay at Pleasant Hills turn into stone when we decide to leave. Down to the very last detail they prove extremely difficult to work with as I try to change the mailing address, stop the phone, the newspaper, cable, and rent. Anything I ask them to do is an effort on their part.

I work within a very small framework of time, six weeks to be exact. This is because Mom's 100 days in rehab are dwindling and I want to avoid moving Mom back in with Dad if I possibly can. As long as she is already separated from him, I think it will be less of a concern if she doesn't temporarily go back to their apartment and then go into her own new facility in Denver. Their current contract specifies that they must give a month's notice before their fees can be suspended. Since we are already into April, I will need to pay their rent for May in both their old and new places.

How Will They Get to Denver?

After the housing arrangements are finalized and the contracts read and signed and the paperwork filled out, I move to the next item on my agenda: getting them from Chicago to Denver. Again, as a beginning, I go to my friend, the internet. Of course, my first choice is to hire a private plane and nurse! The cost of that service is around $10,000! Cross out that choice.

Then there is the possibility of driving from Chicago to Denver in a van. Takes too long and costs too much.

I call the airlines to find out what kind of arrangements they can make for transporting the elderly and the disabled. My query leads to nothing except I can order a wheelchair for each one of them. According to the airlines, no preference can be made for reserving a seat near a restroom or at the front of the plane.

Thinking that purchasing first class or business class tickets might be the answer, I inquire and discover that each seat is priced at well over $1,000. I guess I could handle this, but I keep thinking there must be a better solution.

Finally I ask the facility where my parents are still living if they have any suggestions. Fortuitously they are able to recommend a company that is owned by a nurse who makes your plane reservations, orders oxygen for the travelers, and sends along a nurse to watch over the individual, all for around $3,000. SOLD! It isn't the easiest arrangement I ever make, but I am grateful for the service they offer and cross my fingers that it will work out. There is a tremendous amount of back and forth and a lot of waiting while the tickets are purchased for my mom, my dad, the nurse and me. There are more papers to sign, mostly releases and, of course, more down payments. I write the checks from my own account. I figure I can settle up with my dad later.

Planning the Move

From Denver I contact movers from Move 'Em, the same company that had originally packed and moved Mom and Dad to Pleasant Hills. I make arrangements for them to do all of the packing the day before the move and to hire a long distance mover to transport the furniture and other belongings to Denver. The company also suggests a local charity that will pick up the remainder of the furniture and another company to take some of the remaining furniture on a consignment basis. I coordinate all of these arrangements on the phone from Denver.

In the meantime, my brother and sister-in-law try to get things in order on their home front, i.e. getting Dad organized and making arrangements for Dad to sell his car. Dad continues to throw out every paper he doesn't feel is absolutely necessary to take with him. This turns out to be a great void for me when he arrives in Denver. Amazingly he does save all the basic papers that I will need to work with. In between his tasks, he dines with friends and plays bridge and says good-by to those who have been his support system for the last 50 years.

My father had been going through his personal belongings for quite a while. They say as you get older you start giving things away. He had wanted to give his caregiver his house before we talked him out of this. Then he started to throw away pictures, which we tried to salvage. Luckily my niece is able to save some of the photos. He gives away several of his treasured gold filigree bound Jewish books to his beloved synagogue and all of his old thirty three and a third record albums to his financial planner, a serious collector.

Mom Is Temporarily Rejected from Oak Tree

The nurse at Oak Tree, Mom and Dad's new Denver residence, called today.

"Your mom does not 'qualify' for a temporary assisted living apartment even with a caregiver. She will have to wait for a space in the dementia unit some place else."

I am panicked. This first "glitch" should have been a cue for me to realize how these big corporations work. Instead of phoning the executive director and putting the onus on her to figure out what to do, I take it all on myself. I go to my friend the internet to find some temporary place for Mom. No way is she going to live with us. That is out of the question. I guess I'm just not a very warm and fuzzy child.

I look for the closest dementia unit within the corporate system that my parents are now a part of and find one in a nearby suburb that I can get to in about twenty minutes in good traffic and about forty-five minutes during rush hour. I tell them my sob story and they actually feel sorry for me. They have a space for Mom. I meet the acting executive director and the activities director for the dementia unit. They are so caring and supportive that, even though the facility is not as "plush," seems like it will take very good care of Mom. And really, what choice do I have? I guess I can look some more. I veto that idea and live with my decision.

While I am visiting the temporary unit I spot a familiar face, an elderly and attractive resident. She is the mother of an old friend whom I have not seen in a long time. It comforts me to know that Mom will be living in the same place where someone that I know is residing.

Again, I fill out all the paperwork. This time it goes faster because I know the drill and, thank goodness, I have made copies of the information that I had filled out the first time.

I thank every god I can think of that this works out. All I have to do is redirect the movers.

Memo To Family

Here's the plan:

Friday, April 29th - Mimi to Chicago

Wednesday, May 4th
          6:00 pm - Keith (my husband) and Steve (our son) deliver furniture to Cherry Knolls (Mom's temporary residence).

Thursday, May 5th

    10:36 am - Mom, Dad, Mimi and Nurse Elaine arrive at DIA (United #0245, leaves at 8:53 am)

    11:00 am - Keith and Jen (our daughter-in-law) and our new grandbaby Jude arrive in two cars at passenger pick-up

    We will need to pick up Mom's, Dad's and my luggage. We will all go directly to Cherry Knolls where they have set up lunch for us in a separate dining room. A caregiver (for Mom) will meet us at Cherry Knolls.

    1:30 pm - Nurse Elaine leaves Cherry Knolls by car or taxi for the airport

    3:59 pm - Nurse Elaine's return flight departs

Call me if you have any questions. I love you all especially for helping to make this happen.

Packing up the Packrats

I have arrived in Chicago and am getting ready to move Mom and Dad. Every minute is accounted for.

As usual, I stay at the nearby Hampton Inn where I know all the help and where I can escape every night with a bottle of wine and watch my cable news shows. As usual, I rent a car. This, I note to myself, will be the last time that I will perform a routine that has been a part of my husband's and my lives for the past ten years we have visited my parents and could no longer stay with them. This time I am on my own and my husband is on duty at the other end with my son and daughter-in-law as back ups to be there when we arrive in Denver.

The week has a fully packed agenda.

The first thing I do is take out all of Mom's valuables and collectibles and place them on the dining room table and on the windowsills that surround the table. This includes a huge blue and white china collection, all of her silver pieces and embroidered linens that she had brought with her from Germany in 1938, her extensive jewelry collection, and a more limited Native American art collection that she has accumulated from my past southwestern gallery and from her trips to the Southwest. Luckily before Mom lost her speech, she had spent one memorable evening with me on a prior visit and had made me write down what pieces of jewelry she wanted to give each of us.

All of the Chicago family also goes through the remains of the collectibles as well as the myriad of paintings and artwork and select what they want. On long distance phone calls with my kids, I ask them what they want too. Everything I select can be packed up and sent with the movers and then delivered to our Denver house. My brother and sister-in-law just keep loading up their car and taking items back to their nearby home.

I meet with the consignment lady and we tag all of the pieces that will be picked up by a moving company on the same day the national movers appear. A charity has been contracted to take away the remaining furniture on moving day.

All of the household items, i.e. dishes, pots and pans, appliances, and linens are separated as well. The basics are packed up and are marked to send to Denver for Dad's apartment and the remaining items that no one claims are taken to the nearby Hadassah (the Jewish equivalent of Goodwill) outlet.

My Dad is totally disoriented. He runs around asking, "What do you want me to do?" I tell him to take care of sorting out his clothes. "You need two sport coats, one for summer and one for winter. You need two weeks worth of shirts and underwear. You need two pairs of good pants, one for summer and one for winter. You need two suits." He gets sidetracked with some kitchen items that need to be decided upon, and I try as patiently as possible to refocus him. I ask him to choose a handful of sweaters from the more than three dozen that are housed in his bureau. Most of them all look alike anyway so it doesn't really make any difference which ones he selects. I tell him to select three pairs of gloves and three scarves and to whittle down his sock collection to fit in one drawer rather than three. Then it's time to tackle the coats. "You can only take one leather jacket," I tell him. (He has three!)

My mother's closet contains triple the amount of inventory as Dad's.

To this day, my most vivid memory of Mom and Dad's move is a picture of Mom's discarded clothing stacked in a pile that was taller than my five foot height and that I then needed to pack up in plastic bags and take to rummage. I could not believe how many suits, skirts, dresses, shirts, blouses, purses, and shoes we gave away and how much remained in the closet ready to be packed for Denver!!!! If I had not kept hauling off the bags, I would not have been able to walk around the entire bedroom.

One of my mom's friends helps me pack up some of the items and accompanies me on several of the trips I make to the Hadassah outlet. It is lovely having her company and support.

My mother remains downstairs in the nursing unit with the caregiver oblivious to all the preparations being made. She does know she is moving to Denver. I'm not sure who tells her, but I think my brother tells her some weeks before. With her it is never really clear what she does and doesn't know is going on.

Though I have done most of the paperwork releasing Mom and Dad from Pleasant Hills, there are still some final arrangements to be made. I set up a conference with the director. She lectures and rants about the Comcast boxes but gives us no indication on other things like mail and withdrawal of funds. I foresee trouble.

My dad has sold his car to my brother's friend's son and the transfer takes place a few days before we leave. I think this is hardest for Dad. He loves that Buick, but he seems to be glad to know where it will be going. He makes sure his new owner understands all the ins and outs of the vehicle before he hands him the keys.

In Denver my husband and my son move a bed and a television and a few other pieces of furniture into Mom's temporary unit a few days before we board the plane for Denver.

Then it's time to make the final preparations.

The Movers Arrive

The packers have arrived. It's been a struggle occupying Dad while they're working.

I have packed enough clothes for Mom and for Dad to take on the plane and to last for the ten days it will take for the movers to deliver the remaining clothes and furniture to Denver. The movers will make two stops in Denver. They will take Dad's clothes and furniture to Dad's new apartment in Oak Tree and the remaining furniture and boxes to our house. I have marked all items accordingly.

The night before we leave, my brother and his family and Dad and I go out to dinner at one of our usual "joints." It is a bittersweet evening that needs to end early because the flight the next morning will be very early.

The Journey

Nurse Elaine, who will be traveling with us, arrives at 6:00 am on the morning of the move. She has blonde curly hair and is a bit buxom. She is wearing a white nurse's pant outfit so we'll always know what her role is. She is breezy and funny and totally at ease as she maneuvers around Mom's unit to help Annie get Mom ready. We have asked the nursing facility at Pleasant Hills to feed Mom breakfast and, of course, they say 6:00 am is too early, so my brother goes to McDonald's and gets both Dad and Mom some breakfast. Dad comes downstairs to be with Mom and then my brother and I wheel Mom out to the car in her new wheelchair that the nurse's company has purchased through Medicare. After we put Mom and Nurse Elaine and some of the luggage into my brother's car, my brother takes off for the airport. Soon after they depart, Dad and I climb into the rental car with the remainder of the luggage and head for the same destination. My sister-in-law stays behind at the apartment to supervise the movers and charity and consignment pick-ups that have been arranged.

I drop Dad off at departures where he meets up with my brother, the nurse and my mom. While I am returning the rental car, my brother says his good-byes to our parents and leaves them with Nurse Elaine who is adjusting the oxygen tanks on Mom and Dad's wheelchairs and helping them to get comfortable. I return the rental car, and then catch up with our group and the four of us then head for the concourse and on to Denver.

We sit two and two on opposite sides of the airplane in the first row of the coach section, a feat I'm still trying to figure out how the company I used was able to arrange. My dad and I sit on one side and Nurse Elaine and Mom on the other. We wave back and forth continually. There are lots of smiles. Nurse Elaine is in deep discussion with Mom pointing out the activities taking place on the tarmac. Mom looks on with pleasure. This is a big adventure, and though my parents are in their nineties, they still love an adventure.

One hour and forty-five minutes later we arrive in Denver and are met at the airport by my husband and my daughter-in-law and my two-month-old grandson! We need two cars to hold us all. We load Mom's, Dad's and my luggage into one or the other car, and when we are all packed up, we head to Mom's new temporary home where they welcome us with a lunch in their private dining room. Though the tuna fish sandwich is worse than Mom's and though our new grandson cries through it all, it is reassuring to be together and to have the major move over. It is a pleasant reminder to Mom and Dad that, even though it is sad that they are leaving their familiar home, they will have a new support system

After lunch, my daughter-in-law and the baby go home. We wait for Mom's temporary caregiver to arrive. Then we leave Mom on her own and go back to our house, drop Dad and me off, and my husband takes the nurse to the airport. After Dad is comfortably situated, I return to Mom's new place to make sure Mom is OK. She seems just fine. In fact as she gets ready to go to dinner, she looks around for her lipstick, which she finds in her purse with the help of the caregiver. I return to our house to try to establish a routine for the next ten days that Dad will be our houseguest and for Mom and Dad's new life to begin in Denver.

Note to self: Take a deep breath. You did it. For better or worse, they are here with you in Denver.

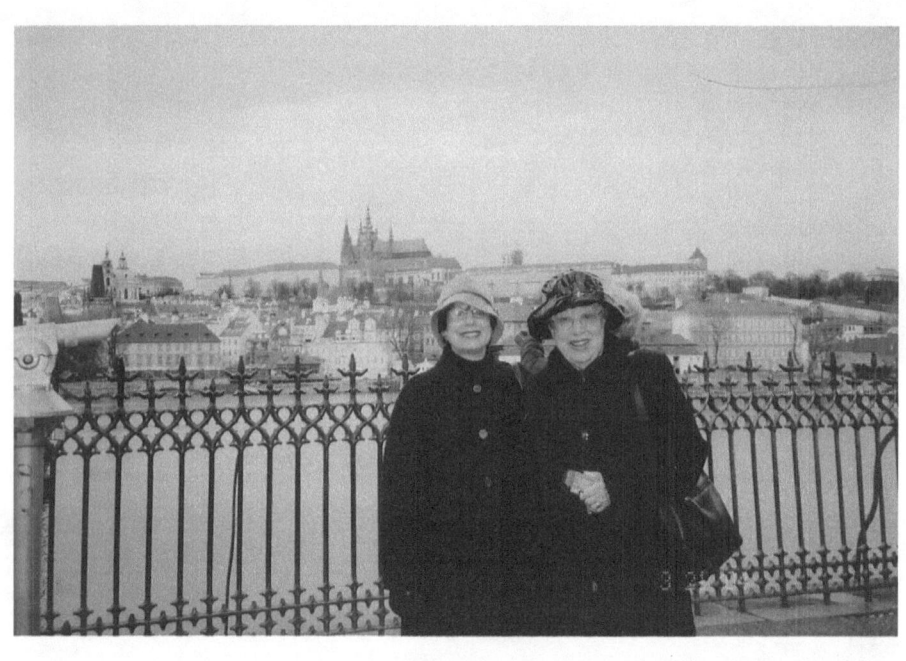

Chapter Eight

Settling In

My family has just expanded to include two more people. I need four more hours in the day!

May 2011

The First Few Weeks

We are going through an adjustment period. My parents must first live in new and foreign temporary surroundings and then move on to their more permanent and again new quarters. My family has to find extra time to include them in their lives. My husband has to get used to faster meals and more time with my father, and I have to try and find ways to keep my same schedule with two extra people to manage and oversee.

Dad is staying with us for ten days until his furniture arrives, and Mom is in a temporary situation until Oak Tree can find a permanent spot for her. It's a challenge to keep everyone on an even keel. I just plunge ahead and hope for the best. I think the newness has some sort of appeal for Mom and Dad. Our kids and grandkids do not have difficulty maintaining their busy schedules. Probably my husband feels the most jarred since my dad has taken over his bedroom and his recliner in the den. For me, if I can just get through the day, find some clean clothes and get in a little exercise, I'm happy or else maybe just numb.

Mothers' Day

For the first time since Mom and Dad have arrived in Denver, I have a brunch at our house to celebrate Mothers' Day. We pick up Dad, Mom and a caregiver and bring them all to the house where we are joined by our children and grandchildren. We dine on lox and bagels and eggs and exchange gifts. It's lovely having four generations together.

MOM

My mom has adjusted to her temporary dementia unit without too many incidents. I hire extra caregivers for her for the first several days until Mom is totally acclimated to her new surroundings. Each caregiver has certain requirements that they think are important like making sure we have rubber gloves and handiwipes in the room, enough hangers, and food for the refrigerator. I run out and make the purchases. They also send me out to buy Thicket to add to Mom's liquids. She is prone to choking. Despite their continuing demands, Mom has fallen down in the bathroom while two caregivers were in attendance.

I am using the doctor's services at the facility where she is staying. It takes a while to meet her. Every day someone different shows up, and the only time I ever get any one's attention is if I take the elevator upstairs and talk to whoever is on duty. Mostly that turns out to be a nurse, never the same nurse, and most likely a new nurse. The doctor somehow always seems to appear when I'm not around, and she never calls to talk to me. I hear about her concerns days later. The time frame is in slow motion. The only thing that's important to the nurse assistants and the nurse is getting the medications distributed to the residents on time. It reminds me of our cleaning lady. She only cares about folding the toilet paper in the bathrooms! Forget about scrubbing the corners on the floor.

The regular caregivers who are in charge at the dementia unit also have their own routines. Given they have no visible supervisor, they are perfectly comfortable making their own rules. On their own terms, they dress and undress Mom each day, take her to the bathroom, usher her into the dining room for meals and occasionally try to encourage her to participate in the activities they now and then organize. They regularly bathe Mom and do her laundry. In this kind of environment, every resident has to speak up about her needs or she gets no attention. And, of course, my mom can't speak, but that never keeps her from making her needs known. She is perfectly content to raise her hand and wave it until someone acknowledges her.

Of course, in a dementia unit, a visitor must ring a bell or knock or scream or yell or go to the receptionist's desk in order for someone to come

The Takeover

and let you in. Especially when one is trying to deliver necessities or supplies, this system can be a bit cumbersome.

The clothes that I have packed for Mom to wear until the movers arrive turn out to be inappropriate. It's a lot warmer in Denver in May than it is in Chicago and Mom's clothes are way too heavy. I make a trip to our local Target to fill in the void in Mom's wardrobe, and that seems to offset that particular issue.

I have eliminated the caregivers I hired for the first few days. They really don't do much for Mom. She seems to be capable of attending to her own needs more than we have given her credit for. The regular caregivers for the most part are enough to get her through the day. My own feeling is that she likes having a little more independence. Though at the beginning she seemed to have fallen more frequently, now that she has relaxed a little, she appears to have become acclimated to her new environment, and her falls have lessened. The unit is still required to call me every time Mom falls. They also have to call when she becomes aggressive, a pattern that continues to exist. The unit's policy is to send the patient to the Emergency Room in either case. Luckily the unit is somewhat flexible on this policy and Mom hasn't been sent out so far.

The light of Mom's life is Brad, her activities director. Brad is in his early thirties. He wears glasses and has a goatee and he looks just like all the thirty-something people you would meet at a Denver brewery. He's just very down to earth. He takes his job very seriously and he is entirely dedicated to making sure everyone in the unit is taken care of and that they are participating in whatever activity he may be offering. During the day he seems to be in charge, and when he is there, I always feel better.

Brad has suggested getting a walker for Mom. Up until now, she has tried unsuccessfully to use a cane, and we have never entertained the idea of purchasing a walker. Almost immediately I run out to the nearest Walgreen's. Of course I mull over all the options without a clue as to which choice is best. I decide on a maroon colored one (it's the prettiest) and it has a nice box where you can put things you might want to bring with you when you are out and about. It takes Mom only a minute to buy into the idea. In no time at all she whizzes around her premises. Wherever she lands, she finds a chair and then she props her feet up on the seat of the walker and watches the world go by.

Brad has begun to involve Mom in all of the activities that are occurring. Today they've been playing Wii bowling. When I come in, he can't wait to talk to me. "Wait until you see Liese," he reports enthusiastically. Then he recreates the morning session and Mom shows off her skills at bowling which in the past were very good. I love Brad. Mom responds so beautifully to him. I don't think I ever saw her smile like that when she lived in Chicago. I think some of this has to do with the fact that he is a man and Mom, who adored her father, has always looked up to male figures. I think she likes him too because he is such an upbeat, positive person. With him around, there is always something good going on.

Mom's room seems very comfortable. She looks out on a patio where we have been taking lots of walks.

I go to see Mom every day and sometimes Dad comes with me. He only has patience to see her for short periods of time. He always says, "She doesn't know me," but when Mom sees Dad she always reaches out her hand to him. In a few minutes he is ready to sit out in the lobby while I tidy up Mom's room and see what she's missing. The dementia unit is not for Dad. He doesn't mind, though, taking Mom for a walk out on the patio. There's a swing there where he and Mom occasionally sit together. I like that.

The residents are very colorful. One woman never stops talking to you and monopolizes every caregiver in the unit. It seems like everywhere I go, she's there! Most of the others obediently follow the suggestions to do whatever is going on in the common area. My friend's mom locks herself up in her room and never comes out except to eat. Mom is selective, but she doesn't seem unhappy. I think she's just glad to be up and about rather than confined to a double occupancy room in a nursing unit. As has always been true for her entire life, her favorite time of day is mealtime. Every caregiver reports to me that she "eats well."

DAD

My husband and I have shifted our sleeping quarters to the upstairs and allocated our first floor master bedroom to Dad. He seems to sleep well in our bed. We try to work him into our routines. We've been on walks with him, to the Farmers' Market and out to dinner. He loves evaluating the restaurants and trying new ones. During the day he happily occupies my husband's recliner in the den and watches lots of ballgames.

We have taken him to see his new quarters where he will be permanently living once his furniture arrives. His apartment is on the 16th floor (it is the only one available and $500 more a month from the base rate because it is on a higher floor). It is an airy apartment with beautiful views. A small patio opens out from the living room. He wants to know the exact distance from our house to his. It takes several days of reassurance before he believes that he only lives a couple of miles away from us.

We show him the bar and the dining room and he walks into the dining room to scout it all out. Quickly he steps out of the room and declares, "These are not my people!"

We aren't sure what that means. Does it mean that there aren't enough Jewish people there? (The place has a good representation of Jewish people.) Does it mean that they don't look like people from Chicago? (I remember feeling the same way when I first moved to Denver thirty years before.)

I think I've almost got Dad set up. We've been to the bank and transferred his account to Denver. We went to Verizon to update his cell phone. We've gone to Walgreen's to get him his favorite kind of Depends and his Polident.

MIMI

It's taking a while to get used to this new title of caregiver. I know I'm a wife, a mother and a grandmother. I know I need to work out, take care of myself, do my household chores, have some fun and occasionally try to write, but I'm trying to figure out how to make this all happen and add on the new task of returning to being a daughter but this time tending to my parents instead of them tending to me.

To Do List for Week of June 6th:

1) Wash Mom's bathmat. Make sure it's the right size
2) Call Mom and Dad's friend Ethel
3) Call Dad's cousin Nora
4) Go to cleaners
5) Call vet about our dog
6) Look into drip in master bath in Denver house
7) E-mail my daughter-in-law's mother
8) Check noise in crawl space for critters
9) Buy grandson jeans, dinosaur pjs and slippers
10) Talk to daughter-in-law's brother re taking some of Mom and Dad's furniture (He has recently separated from his wife)
11) Hairdresser appointment
12) Make bone density appointment
13) Office supplies
14) Schedule summer concerts
15) Alarm and handyman
16) Call my son's in-laws
17) Contact Meredith (my grammar school girlfriend who will be coming to Denver to visit her son who lives here.)

I have bought myself an orange star plant for Mother's Day. I am enjoying watching it grow, watering it (probably too much) and trying to figure out why the leaves are starting to turn yellow. I move it around to see if the light makes a difference.

I thrive on Morning Joe and the Today Show. Yesterday Willard Scott looked pretty tired, like he's lost all his pep when he shows all those centenarians. There was one guy on the Smuckers special who was 105. That would mean ten more years that Dad would still be living and fifteen more for Mom. Yikes, the money's going to run out.

It's been raining all day today. Along with my chores of taking grandkids to school and shopping for supplies for Dad at the Safeway, I have spent five hours talking and visiting with the post office, my parents' former residence director, and my sister-in-law in Chicago. It seems that my parents' mail is not being delivered to their new addresses. Selma, Pleasant Hills' resident manager, pleads innocence in the whole manner and I learn to work around her. I am totally upset with the lack of interest on all ends. Finally I get my sister-in-law to pick up my parents' month's worth of mail and send it to Denver. Then I contact the Chicago post office and direct them on how to forward the mail from Pleasant Hills. Finally I fill out forms at the post office in Denver and then for several days afterward I check to make sure an effective system has been established.

On a recent Saturday, my husband, Dad and I attended a family barbeque at Mom's dementia unit. The food was surprisingly good and the mood festive. The staff circulated and visited with the families and the residents. It was nice to see again my old friend whose mother is also a resident. We tried to stay for a lecture on Alzheimer's Disease, but didn't quite make it. It would have been difficult for us to relate to the discussion since Mom has primary progressive aphasia, a different form of dementia from Alzheimer's disease.

Last night I begged off going to our favorite local hangout for dinner with the children. We rescheduled for Thursday. I drank lots of wine, ate popcorn and fell into a very deep sleep for ten glorious hours. It was the first night I had not worried about my parents since Mom had fallen in Chicago in March.

I have begun to focus on my normal life, i.e. how to help potty train our older grandson, and how to tackle all my currrent household chores. This week our grandson is off from school and I am on extra grandmother duty.

Dad Moves to Oak Tree

The moving truck has arrived today and dropped off the furniture at Dad's new place. I have made Dad stay at the house while I have directed the movers on where to place the furniture. I have tried to create an environment that is more for Dad than for Mom, sort of an elderly "man cave." My husband has come over to Oak Tree to hang some of the pictures we sent from Chicago. I arrange his books on a bookshelf, hook up his computer on his desk, and set all kinds of family pictures around. I make the beds and in his bathroom I hang a new shower curtain that matches the bedspreads in his bedroom. I bring over some old wicker chairs from our house to place on the patio so that Dad can enjoy the view.

Dad is thrilled with his apartment. What is not to like when you are on the 16th floor and you have a beautiful mountain view from your own patio?

"Wow!" He says as he surveys all his belongings cozily set in his new "digs."

"How did you do this?" he asks in wonderment. I think to myself that I'm not sure how I did this, but thank goodness it's done.

We go downstairs to dine, and then my husband and I say good night and leave him for the first time. It is almost like the day when we dropped off our children for their first night at college.

It is taking a while for Dad to get completely set up. We are having trouble connecting the television. We call in Oak Tree's handyman who looks like a leprechaun. He tinkers with the television for a few minutes and then declares, "You should buy a new one." Dad says he doesn't need a TV. I'm pretty sure the house handyman has not pursued all possible avenues, so I call Sony and then for a couple of hours we go through the process of starting up the TV. We manage to do this despite the fact that we seem to have lost the remote. Sony promises to send us a new one. Months later, we find the original remote!

The next day I get a call from Dad asking when the Bulls game comes on. Do I think he doesn't need a TV?

After Dad settles in, we make our virgin trip to the grocery store for some serious shopping. I try to encourage him to use one of the electric carts and he refuses. The session takes over an hour as we go down each aisle selecting orange juice, coffee, milk, eggs, herring and the rest of his shopping list. Then we update his Safeway card and eventually check out. I make Dad pay. He's got to get used to fending for himself. I don't know about Dad, but I need a nap!

Dad's easy chair had seen its better days so on the weekend after the move, my dad, my husband and I go out shopping for a new chair, my husband's and my housewarming gift to Dad. What a hoot! Dad hasn't been to a massive furniture warehouse probably ever but in at least twenty-five years. He tries out all the recliners that appeal to him, pays careful attention to the prices and finally selects a soft beige cushioned one that seems to fit his small frame perfectly. They deliver it the next week and he is now happily ensconced in it almost every time I come to visit.

Two doctors are associated with the senior facility where Dad is living and Mom will eventually live and both are geriatricians. I have arbitrarily hired one of them to be the doctor for Dad and who can also take care of Mom as well when she moves to Oak Tree. This requires more paperwork. The nice thing about the doctor being tied to the facility where they reside is that he or a member of his staff is in the building every Friday. We make an appointment to meet Dr. Higby for the first Friday that Dad is in the building. He appears promptly. Dr. Higby is in his late fifties. He has white hair, a well trimmed gray beard and he wears a crisp white doctor's coat. He carries his doctors' case and makes copious notes on his I-Pad as he examines Dad. He speaks very slowly and respectfully to Dad and peppers his conversation with all kinds of anecdotes and observations. He teaches part-time at the University of Denver and he has a professorial demeanor. He takes his time, the direct opposite approach to Mom and Dad's Chicago doctor who was always in a hurry. Of course after Dad meets Dr. Higby, he sizes him up immediately and declares that he is an "**!" I have already learned to ignore both of my parents' assessments of anybody. (Mom never liked our Chicago caregiver). I have to make a choice on everyone and if I listen to my parents and change every time they complain and then start over again, it is hard for me to focus and move forward. To me Dr. Higby seems perfectly charming. I know Oak Tree would not have contracted him if he wasn't well respected and I have also looked him up on the internet just to check him out.

At first Dad wants to dine with my husband and I each night, and at first I want to dine with him each night. Sandra, the dining director is always happy to see Dad. "Hello Mr. Rothman," she'll chant. Then she'll speak to my husband and I and report her efforts to try and get Dad to dine with some other people when we're not there. Dad, as usual, is not cooperative and eventually settles into a routine of dining downstairs by himself unless my husband and I join him. He eats his breakfast and lunch in his apartment.

Dad has looked into going grocery shopping on one of Oak Tree's scheduled visits to the grocery store. After one expedition, he allocates that responsibility to me.

I don't think he likes making lists and planning ahead. Basically I have been placed in charge of the grocery shopping and the laundry. (I choose to do the laundry to absorb the extra charge of paying for Dad's more expensive rent on a higher floor in the building.)

Dad Takes a Spill

Dad has gone walking around the neighborhood and has taken a nasty spill. He didn't tell anyone. We had picked him up so we could visit our son and daughter-in-law and it was only when we got to the house that our daughter-in-law, a doctor's daughter, discovered his wounds and cleaned and bandaged him up. Apparently he got lost circling the block around the building. A lecture from me has followed about how he should not walk alone. I have since created identification cards for both him and Mom. I have instructed Dad to put the card in his wallet in case of any other incidents. We were fortunate that someone came and helped him up and directed him back to his residence.

Mom Moves to Oak Tree

It's now been almost a month since we settled Dad into his new residence. We have received a call saying that an apartment in the dementia unit in Dad's building has become available. The marketing person has been kind enough to push Mom's name to the top of the list. I think she realizes that I am commuting back and forth between parents and that the commute down to see Mom is a good half hour more than the five minute one to Dad's place. During rush hour, that half hour commute has been taking even longer.

I have mixed feelings about transferring Mom. She has settled into a routine and is doing reasonably well at her temporary quarters. We need to be pragmatic though and so I begin to orchestrate her move.

When we had moved Dad into his place, we had met a local mover on the elevator. He had given my husband his card and so we called him up and asked him to help us move Mom's furniture and clothes to her new facility and to pick up the other furniture at her temporary apartment. At this point my husband and son were only too happy to relinquish their moving responsibilities. After all, they have day jobs too. We now have an official mover that becomes our "go to" person every time another move is made and there will be several more!!!

Mom's permanent furniture that we have stored in our basement is delivered first. Mom's new quarters are as lovely as Dad's. We furnish it with her favorite gold chair and ottoman, her lovely blue and white embroidered antique chair and her blue and white barrel chair. I have even found a blue and white shower curtain at Target (it is pricey, but I pay for it myself) to hang in her bathroom. We have to put the bed very near the bathroom since she has to go quite frequently. We have given Dad the fancy Dux beds for his apartment because they fill up the bedroom. Mom's bed just has a metal frame. We place her oak library table on one end of the bed and another table lamp between the two chairs. Again, my husband hangs some of their pictures that have been transported from Chicago to Denver. Mom cannot have any glass or breakables in her apartment but we work around that rule and the place in our mind looks great. I hang all her clothes in her closet and place her other clothes in her own mahogany dresser drawer that she has owned for more than fifty years. Though I can't bring any of her good jewelry to her new place, I string a dozen or so of her beads from her extensive collection on hangars in her closet so that she still feels like she can get dressed up. I make up the bed with a new comforter that I have purchased to match the color scheme. She is set to go.

We pick up Mom and wheel her out in her wheelchair and carry along her walker and her suitcase. Then the mover comes in and moves the television and the rest of the furniture.

Finally Mom and Dad are both at the same residence. I miss the devotion paid to Mom by her activities director, but I don't miss the commute. Certainly the new facility is much more elegant. She seems to have accepted the move without too much objection.

At no time during all of Mom's and Dad's moves does the Oak Tree administration do much in the way to help us. They always send a gift basket full of stuff that you would never want to eat, but whoever is on duty does the welcoming and believe me, it isn't much. One thing I learn about the attitude of the place where they live is that they all take a "business as usual" approach and I believe this is intentional. Any disturbance to daily life is invasive to the residents. If one can believe that moving in and moving out is normal and that visits from the paramedics is a regularly occurring activity, everyone is much better off than they would be if a big deal was made of anything.

For Mom's new move, I again hire extra caregivers for the first few days until she gets used to things. She seems to be adjusting fairly well. I go up to visit her and sometimes Dad comes too. It is so nice having both of them in the same place. Heidi, the program director warmly invites Dad to come often and have a snack and enjoy the afternoon entertainment and Dad is very receptive. Like Mom enjoyed Brad, Dad is totally enchanted by the fair-haired Heidi.

A week after her move, Mom develops congestion in her lungs. The doctor who visits Oak Tree every Friday drops in to make sure that she is OK.

Some Sort of Normalcy

My daily schedule now involves my regular routine of exercising, running errands, taking care of grandchildren and preparing dinners as well as tending to Mom and Dad's needs.

Most of the medical concerns seem to be under control for the moment. When Mom arrived, Dr. Higby paid her a visit. He has now visited with both Mom and Dad and periodically stops in on Fridays to see how they are doing.

Tiffany at Oak Tree's Home Health department has contacted me about getting Mom and Dad enrolled in the program they offer. She brusquely explains to me how the system works. She tells me that under Medicare seniors are entitled to a number of physical and occupational therapy sessions if they sign up for the program. Once those sessions have been completed, they can continue the program by paying a relatively inexpensive copayment. Tiffany makes it sound like it's just a common assumption that anyone would want this service. I decide that we have nothing to lose, so I sign both Mom and Dad up for the program. I visit the department to fill out the paperwork. Several desks line the outer office, the most expansive being Tiffany's. She is not a therapist, but rather she is a clerk of some sort who schedules therapists with the residents and takes care of reporting to Medicare who then pays Oak Tree's staff for their services. The small inner office is the "physical therapy room" equipped with a limited number of machines and weights to work with residents who hire the department's services.

The therapists show up to both Mom's and Dad's when they feel like it. They never communicate with me and they always seem to appear at odd times of the day such as when Dad naps or during the afternoon activity sessions at Elm Place that Mom so enjoys. What a system!!! There are some good parts. Dad is learning how to use a calendar and how to orient himself to the facilities available to him at Oak Tree. Mom is getting some help in learning how to go to the bathroom and how to get in and out of chairs. It's just so disorganized.

Memorial Day

The children come with the grandkids to see Mom and Dad. The boys prance down the halls of Oak Tree and find them in the main living area listening to Heidi, the activities director, talk about Memorial Day. Mom is seated on her walker and is fast asleep until we all get there.

After we visit Mom, Dad and the whole family go downstairs to a sumptuous buffet. It's a family affair.

Note to self: Take things in stride. We're making progress. It just doesn't always seem that way.

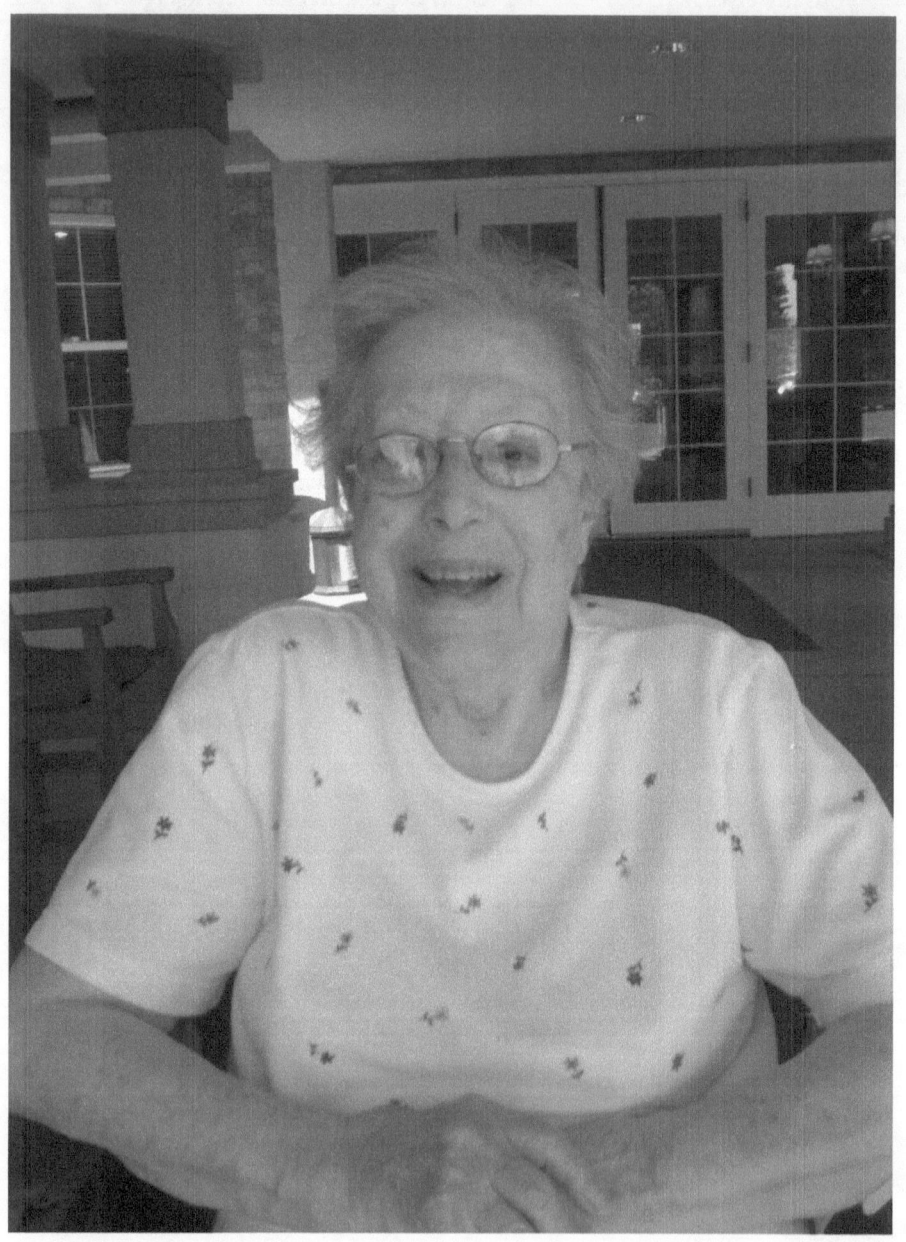

Chapter Nine

Mom's World

I love Mom's spirit. She's got a lot of issues, but she's a fighter.

June 2011

I Want to Go Home

The first time I go to see Mom after we have transferred her from her temporary quarters to her new permanent facility my husband and I push the buzzer and are let in by one of the staff members. We find her in one of the anterooms off the reception area. She is sitting in a chair with her walker next to her. We bend down to greet her (we have learned that one needs to speak at eye level) and then we pull up chairs to keep her company.) She takes my hand and, though she can hardly speak, she blurts out what she is feeling. "I want to go home," she says quite clearly.

She doesn't know that she's breaking my heart.

I hold her hand and I say, "Mom, I wish you could go home, but we can't take care of you there anymore, so this is your new home. And we're going to try very hard to make it as happy as we can for you here. We're going to come and visit you all the time and Dad is nearby and he'll visit you too."

After that day she never complains again and with her incredible ability to adapt to whatever circumstances are handed to her, she faces her new situation head on and begins to involve herself in her new community. This is a woman who left her home in Germany at the age of eighteen, came to America to escape the Nazis and never again saw her family.

Life at Elm Place

Mom's permanent dementia unit is much more elegant and inviting than the temporary one where she initially stayed, but both units have many things in common. The current unit is much bigger with many different rooms rather than one large room. Various nooks and crannies house games and dolls, stuffed animals, crafts, tools and books. Both places have access to an outdoor patio where residents can sit either with guests or by themselves and where gardening activities occur, but Mom's new place is accessed from the second floor of an eighteen story high rise rather than on a ground floor. There is a very large dining area that doubles for crafts and cooking activities and a living area furnished with comfortable couches and chairs where residents and their families can watch television or gather for the many performance presentations that are brought to them. There is even a piano. Behind the wall is a windowed nurse's station so that the nurse assistants and caregivers can watch the residents at all times. There is a partial kitchen on the premises as well as a beauty salon and laundry facilities.

Normally around eighteen residents at a time live in the unit. Only one of the rooms has double occupancy. The rest are single units. Most of the residents have various forms of Alzheimer's disease.

Something out of the ordinary is usually the norm! A certain resident might be agitated and become extremely vocal. Another resident might be sleeping in someone else's room. Unfamiliar family pictures regularly appear in rooms other than the ones in which they belong.

The staff consists of an activities director and an assistant activities director both of whom are scheduled to be there seven days a week on a rotating basis. A nurse of one kind or another (usually a CNA, i.e. certified nurse assistant) is the administrator for distributing all medications and also the resource if anything out of the ordinary is occurring. There is always a chief nurse who is a licensed nurse practitioner (LNP) on duty for both the dementia unit and the assisted living unit but that office is in another part of the building. Two or three caregivers rotate shifts to handle the personal needs of each resident such as dressing, toileting, and bathing.

Though there is supposed to be some sort of predictable schedule, there seldom is. You can come on a certain day and there might be only two caregivers because one is sick and another at a meeting. Most of the caregivers' schedules are staggered and there is little continuity from day to day. That means it is difficult to find out if your loved one is improving unless the CNA looks at the charts and frequently the caregivers forget to record the day's occurrences except on a very limited basis. There are a few regulars who work the same weekly schedule and who have been in the building for many years, but these veterans are rare and also a treasure.

More caregivers are assigned to the morning and the early evening when the needs of the residents are more labor intensive, but residents will often have to wait their turn, and usually the noisiest are attended to first. Generally speaking, the caregivers are very professional and calm, a trait that is most critical to dementia patients. Caregivers also do all of the laundry of the residents. Those residents with housekeeping instincts (not my mother although she had been a great housekeeper) are often seen at the dining room tables helping to fold the table linens.

One of Mom's caregivers, Ilsa, is from Rumania near where Mom grew up in Germany and she loves speaking German to Mom. "Vee Gates, Liese," she is fond of saying and Mom, though I'm not sure it's registering, nods as if she understands. Ilsa often tells me that she likes to take out books of Germany and look at the pictures together with Mom. I love Ilsa!

The setup is less than perfect, but it has a regular rhythm that seems to suit most of the residents. There is a routine for each day that the residents adhere to: breakfast, a morning activity, lunch, rest, exercise, music, dinner and then another activity after dinner. A monthly schedule is available for all residents' families. It defines the regular activities as well as special activites such as field trips or performances that will take place. Of course, they don't always materialize but it does serve as a guideline if you are planning on visiting. These schedules are also mailed to the residents' families and caregivers so that they can make plans accordingly.

When I was choosing a place for Mom to move, I was attracted to this philosophy. Mom had always been a "doer," and I thought she might go for this kind of structured set-up. I thought this approach would be much better than her past routine of late in which she ate, slept and went to see doctors. The theory of this form of housing is that the residents need to have a steady routine that helps stabilize them and that they should be stimulated as much as possible. In other words, no one is giving up on them. I think it's working for Mom.

Mom is in the ER

Fourteen days after Mom moves to Elm Place at 5:30 in the morning I receive a phone call. I have learned to leave my phone in close range to my bed. Mom has fallen and gashed her head. Which hospital do I want to send her to? I tell them to send her to the hospital nearest to where I live and where I have gone in the past for various treatments and surgeries. I quickly don my workout clothes and rush over to meet Mom. She has arrived in the ambulance and been placed in an ER room a few minutes before I get there. When I arrive, she puts out her hand to me and she doesn't let go for most of the time we are there. Various attendants rush around the room monitoring all her vitals and getting her ready to put stitches (there will be eight of them) in her head. I attempt to get the attention of the doctor in charge without looking impatient, an art that I will continue to cultivate for the entire time I am taking care of my parents. A very important basketball game has occurred the night before and the ER doctor and an associate are busy recalling the highlights of the game. I smile, I coddle, I talk about the game too (my husband is also a big fan) and I use my greatest charms to help move the process along. After the doctor finally visits Mom, there is a long hiatus before anything concrete begins to happen. The staff continues to monitor Mom and even to get her some breakfast. At this point she finally is willing to let go of my hand. I drink several cups of coffee and fret over how this all happened as well as how we're ever going to get out of here.

Finally the wheels start to turn. The anesthesiologist numbs Mom's head, and then the doctor puts in the stitches. After they mend her, we wait for all the final red tape that needs to take place before she can leave, another hour or so. Someone asks me how I want to transport Mom back to her dementia unit. I do not realize that it will cost me $700 out of my own pocket if I opt for an ambulance. Selfishly I really don't want to have to deal with putting her in my car. That decision will teach me a lesson. But it will be a problem in the future as well. From the hospital I arrange for caregivers to tend to Mom until she has stabilized after the incident. Our whole episode probably occurs within a five-hour span.

Once Mom is returned to her unit, she does not get monitored with any extra care by the Elm Place staff, but she adjusts without too much difficulty. The extra caregivers I hire are only there for a day.

I try to talk to the staff to help me figure out why Mom has fallen and how the accident has occurred. No one has much to offer about my concerns. When I put the pieces together, my own assessment centers on the arrangement of her furniture. Her metal bedframe has sharp edges. We decide to switch her bed with one of Dad's that has softer wooden edges. Again we call our mover friend Ed to help us out. We then get rid of the wobbly table that had been placed near one of her chairs. I think too that being in a new place and not yet being comfortable with her new situation probably had something to do with the accident.

On Cruise Control

Since the ER incident Mom has been adjusting nicely to her new home. Yes, there are occasional calls. She fell, she scratched a resident, she punched a caregiver but for the most part she is fine. She likes to ramble down the hallway using her spiffy walker. She seems pretty content to participate in the activities she likes and to just sit in her favorite chair and put up her feet on her walker and snooze if she's not interested. Frequently I'll come and visit her at her table in the dining room and she'll be eating with great gusto. The food is excellent!

On a normal day when I visit Mom she is sitting in a chair near a wall a little away from the main couch with her feet up on her walker and she's taking in all the action. When she sees me she holds out her hand and then I pull up a chair and sit next to her. Sometimes I bring a Chico's or Nordstrom catalog and we look through them together. Sometimes Dad comes with and we all sit together. Sometimes Dad comes alone to visit Mom. The activities director pays a lot of attention to Dad and he enjoys whatever activity they are doing at the time. He'll say "They had a great singer this afternoon." If my schedule doesn't allow me to come until late in the day, I will stop by in my gym clothes either before or after my workout to check in on Mom. She is content with a short visit, anywhere from fifteen to twenty minutes before she seems to get bored with me.

When Dad and I visit in the afternoon, she's always happy to see us, but after a short period of time, she's happy to see us go. That's pretty common, the books say. Dad and I both have no problem with her attitude. It's no different than when she was well. After a while, she tired of us then too!!!!

Mostly when I visit Mom, she seems happy to see me. What I don't like is that after I say hello, she grabs her walker and guides me back to her room where she leads me into her bathroom and encourages me to assist her. I have decided it's time to put my foot down. The next time she does this I grab a caregiver to tell her that Mom has to go the bathroom. After that I tell whoever is on duty when she starts to go into the bathroom if I can't talk her out of going. When she tries to get me to take her, I tell her, "Mom, you don't need to go there. Let's go out in the living room." I think she's getting the point.

One of the activities directors made me feel better the other day when I expressed guilt in not wanting to take her to the bathroom. "You shouldn't have to do that. You pay for us to do it," she said in an understanding manner.

I have learned the stories of many of the residents in the unit. One of them had been a prominent attorney in town. Another was a military officer. A couple that I thought was married turned out not to be so but have developed a budding relationship in the unit. Barbara, the resident who roams from room to room and interchanges everybody's belongings wears a different hat each day. She reminds me of Boo Radley in "To Kill a Mockingbird" and Harriet Stanley, the senile sister in "The Man Who Came to Dinner." Jane is so sweet but she's a mumbler and says a lot of nothings that I learn early just require nodding in response. Then there's darling Gert whose daughters lunch with her regularly because "otherwise she won't eat."

Lois, one of the residents has a very loud voice and a huge presence. Everyday she dresses up with gorgeous clothes and matching jewelry. (I have stopped figuring out how this happens to her and not to Mom.) She needs constant attention from the staff and though her family does not come frequently, she is always asking for them. All of us are happier when a member arrives, even though they stay for a very short time.

One of the activities directors told me about a recent altercation Lois and Mom had. Every resident has the same place in the dining room for every meal. Lois happens to sit at Mom's table. The other day after dinner the activities director was giving Mom a hand massage and Lois started complaining in a loud voice, "When's it my turn?" she whined. Mom turned to the activities director and in a complete sentence uttered, "She's a pain in the neck." This story has tickled me for the past few days. When she could talk, Mom had always been outspoken. Even in this environment she seems to still be able to express herself.

Passing the Time

Mom has shown an interest in painting. In Chicago our son had brought some paints and paper to see if she might like to do some artwork and she had expressed no interest, but now that she is in her new unit, she seems to have taken to the activity. This month Mom has been chosen as the "Artist of the Month."

Every time I visit Mom I try to think of something to do to lengthen my stay. Sometimes it's cleaning out her closet or her dresser. Sometimes it's marking her clothes with a Sharpie. Sometimes it's going out on the patio. Sometimes it's bringing Dad down to visit. Mom is always the happiest during snack time. When Dad or I are there, the staff will always offer a snack to us as well. Sometimes if there's lively music, the activities director will ask Mom to dance. One time she did a version of the can can. She was always musical and limber too, and we're seeing vestiges of her old talent once again.

Occasionally when the weather is good I take Mom for a walk outside. I've only started to have the courage to take her in the wheelchair, down the elevator into the lobby and out of the building onto the sidewalk. The sidewalk is a bit bumpy, but once we're outside in nice weather, it's quite enjoyable to have gone through the hassle.

One of the jobs of the staff is to make sure to interact with the family. My usual time of arrival, no matter how hard I try, is in the afternoon around three or four. That's usually the time when the performers come and that gives us something to do together. Last week the entertainer was a one-man band. He had a harmonica, a pedal for drums and then he strummed on the guitar. Mom and I got to shake the maracas as added percussion. I missed the women's choir a couple of days ago. Just got there too late. They have karaoke now and again but unlike at Pleasant Hills the staff knows the songs to choose. When I went to karaoke with Mom last week, I guess I sang too loud, because they handed me the microphone again. I chose "Sweet Rosie O'Grady" and when I was done, Mom clapped for me. After that one of the male residents who has a lovely voice took over.

On the weekends the activities director will show a musical on Saturday (Last week it was "Music Man" and I loved that) but on Sundays Mom and I avoid the religious show. Heidi always comes over to talk to me and tell me how Mom is doing and what kind of a day she's having. She relates to Mom as a human being and gives her all the dignity she deserves. It's really wonderful to watch. Mostly being in the unit reminds me of my days as a camp counselor.

The staff is very interested in finding out more about Mom. They have learned that Mom was a good cook and that she played the piano. They ask me for some of Mom's soup recipes and even make plans for one of their future activities to be "Cooking With Liese" where Mom's barley soup recipe will be featured. When they cook, she'll do a bit of chopping on the occasion, but Mom really doesn't like to tax herself. That's OK with me. She's earned it.

I bring in one of my old duet piano books to see if Mom and I can play on the piano together. There's not much hope for that. Mom will sit down and touch some of the keys but playing a song is not within her ability. I put the duet book in the music bench.

Today's a good day! I've gone to visit Mom and she's not there. It seems she has gone on a picnic with her unit.

At Elm Place today everyone is in a good mood. The caregivers all crowd around Mom and me. We talk about how so many caregivers' names end in "a:" Ilsa, Tonya, Angela, Maria, Sylvia, Gabriela. It's amazing to me that the group is a United Nations among themselves. They come from places like Nigeria, Eritrea, the Dominican Republic, and from all over America. We talk about nail polish and about manners. I tell them that Mom taught me to only slice butter from one end of the stick. It's fun chatting with my new community of "girls."

I am struck by moments of visiting Mom and actually having a good time. We've sung karaoke together and played the piano together, attempted word puzzles together and visited with some of the other residents together.

Elm Place Style

One day I get a call that Mom has fallen tying her shoes. I had put several pairs of shoes in her closet that we had sent from Chicago but none of them seemed to be just exactly what she needed. There were two sets of sandals that she had always loved. They were easy to slip into, especially when she wore them with socks but they were not that sturdy to walk in. The other shoes were tie shoes and that definitely had to be changed. She could barely put on her shoes, let alone tie them. If we would have let her, she would have spent the whole day trying to tie them and they would still not have been done. I decide she needs shoes with velcro straps that are easier to put on. I bring the first set to the unit and try them on her, but they're too tight. I return them and find a better pair and for the remainder of the time that she is living in the unit, she wears them every day. "She loves those shoes," says one of the caregivers.

I have to get used to Mom not always looking perfect. Even though I take great lengths to coordinate her outfits, inevitably when I come to see her, she's wearing a mismatched outfit. It's possible to see her wearing a turtleneck in the summer even though I've buried the turtlenecks in the bottom drawer of her bureau. I'm thrilled that she often wears a set of the beads that I've sent along. I'm not sure whether it's the caregiver's choice or Mom's but it makes my day. My understanding is that the residents help pick out the clothes, but Mom seems to have lost her fashion designer talent. I have brought pretty plastic hangers for her clothes, but they disappear quickly and are replaced by bent wire hangers. Sometimes her clothes disappear too and when they come back from the laundry, they're frequently misshapen. I'm getting used to the drill.

One of the first caregivers who dressed Mom decided she didn't need to wear a bra. The caregiver was an admitted former hippie and didn't think this item was necessary. I complained to the CNA, and the situation never occurred again. I never saw that caregiver again either.

The beauty shop in the unit is open every Tuesday. Not long after Mom's arrival, I have my first confrontation with Dorothy, the beautician. As she is just wheeling Mom into the shop to get her hair done, I mention that we have not set up any arrangement. Dorothy, a bulky platinum blonde, replies in a nasal twang, "Listen honey, I do what I can do. I just fit her in." Excuse me, I think. Do I just accept her plan or voice my concerns for the fact that I'd like to have some idea of the charges and the dates of service. I try out a response but I am speaking to dead ears. I accept my lot but I'm not happy especially when Dorothy starts complaining about Mom being aggressive with her. If she paid any attention to Mom, she'd know not to schedule her late in the day when "Sundowner's syndrome," a type of behavior that often becomes more heightened as the day goes on, begins to surface. Eventually I just decide to tell Dorothy when I think Mom needs attention and let it go at that. I have even stopped trying to figure out how they're charging and to address the problem once a month when I finally receive a bill. The beautician is not allowed to take tips. What a shame that I can't use that as a lure. Even if I could tip her, she'd probably still respond the same way. Whatever.

Initially I had even purchased Mom's favorite nail polish color and brought it to Dorothy to use, but that went unnoticed as well. Instead of the silver platinum polish my mom has worn for years, I'm mostly seeing a variety of pinks and roses. Often her nails chip the next day and sometimes her nails go unattended for weeks until I call Dorothy's attention to the issue. If this is my biggest problem, I can deal with it.

Medical Matters

Mom's new doctor at Oak Tree is Dr. Higby, the same doctor that takes care of Dad. He has reviewed Mom's medical history and recommended making some adjustments to Mom's list of the more than twenty drugs that she takes daily. Her stay in the ER revealed that the drug she was taking for her heart condition was not working. In the chaos of the move, the level of the medication, which required regular monitoring, had not been addressed and had probably been a factor in saving her life. The doctor has suggested taking her off of this strong drug and eliminating or reducing some of the other drugs. "Though there's a risk in reducing some of the medications," he says, "she won't be as sleepy and she'll have a better quality of life." I instinctively go along with his suggestions but convey this approach to my brother for affirmation. We had both watched Mom live her daily life in a stupor because of all the medications she was taking. We're willing to take the chance.

The home health arm of Oak Tree, Senior Care, has contacted me to have Mom also use their facilities in the same Medicare subsidized manner as Dad. Though I am not sure how frequently they come or what exactly they do, I have noticed improvements in Mom's ability to function, particularly when it comes to going to the bathroom. They have asked me to purchase a container to hold Mom's Depends and I quickly go out and find something that adheres to their specifications. And I gladly pay the extra cost for a special toilet seat that the occupational therapist orders from one of their suppliers that they have an agreement with. Both improvements are very helpful.

The sessions have helped Mom learn to navigate on her own and she has exercised more frequently, but I doubt if it will pay to continue this service after the Medicare runs out. She's already turned down some of the sessions. It could be because they show up at all odd hours of the day, but whatever.

It's not worth continuing. She's just not going to start an exercise program at the age of 90 for the first time in her life.

The Dentist

Mom, at age 90, still has a full set of teeth. Oak Tree has an "in-house" father-son dentist team that you contact if you need some dental services. After you make an appointment, you fill out a lot of paperwork and then on the specified date of the appointment, the dentists' van and either the father or the son show up in the parking lot of Oak Tree. Then by whatever means you can, you get your parent downstairs, and you meet up with the dentist. Today it's Doctor Fairly Senior's turn. "Hello, Mrs. Rothman," he says cheerfully as I roll Mom out to Oak Tree's parking lot. Mom gives him a wide smile. Dr. Fairly then maneuvers Mom's wheelchair onto the van's platform and raises her into his "office." I pace outside in the parking lot and a half hour later, Dr. Fairly opens the van's door, lowers Mom down to the payment and offers an excellent report on her session. The dentist has always been a pleasant experience for Mom. Go figure. He then sees Dad who can walk up the stairs to Dr. Fairly's office on his own. Everything goes smoothly and I am greatly relieved. In my usual compulsive way, I had worried about the whole arrangement.

More Activity?

There's another department of Oak Tree that the staff encourages me to use. It's called "Oak Tree Caregiving Services" and the concept here, another moneymaking enterprise that is independently operated by Oak Tree, is to hire extra caregivers on an hourly basis to service the needs of the individual resident.

I decide to take advantage of their caregiver service and hire someone for an hour or so to take Mom for walks a couple of times a week. Though she has never been much for exercising in the first place, it is another activity. After the activities director tells me the caregivers are showing up during the times when scheduled activities are taking place that Mom enjoys, I decide to discontinue these extra sessions. Mom seems very content without the extra activity. She is very happy going on the weekly field trips and showing up for the unit's afternoon entertainment. That seems to be plenty for her.

Late Summer 2011

I've been getting calls occasionally that Mom has been aggressive and hit one of the caregivers or that she has fallen. The staff is required to let me know but unless she's very aggressive and they can't control her with a sedative, they will just take her vitals and, if she seems to be OK, they won't send her to the ER. It does make me mad that Mom seems to have more aggressive incidents with a couple of the caregivers than she does with any of the others. For example, most of the complaints have been on the weekends with the same caregivers. Though I try to gently suggest having other caregivers take care of Mom, the suggestion comes to deaf ears. The unit has to use the staff they have at that moment, I guess.

September 2011

It's the Jewish High Holy Days, and I have decided to make Mom's famous plum cake (Zwetschgenkuchen) to bring to Elm Place for all the staff and the residents. It's fun to do although I'm not sure Mom realizes what I did. I never get the baking sheet back, but that's OK. I've got many more.

November 2011

It's now November and Heidi, the activities director, has announced that the residents have been practicing every Saturday in readiness for a holiday bell concert. A special guest director has been coming in and practicing with the residents. She has chosen several Christmas carols to perform and has distributed different bells with different notes to each resident. When the director points at the resident, they are supposed to ring their bell and all together the residents' bells will present the selection. The anticipation for the final concert has been building. The concert is sure to be the highlight of the season and of a very busy year for Mom.

Note to self: You must continue to keep working on courting those members of the staff at Elm Place that you can consistently rely on. Though it's hard to figure out who does what, I think that Tina, the assistant activities director, and Jeannie, the certified nurse assistant, are easiest to talk to. Heidi's great too, but she has such a huge responsibility for everyone.

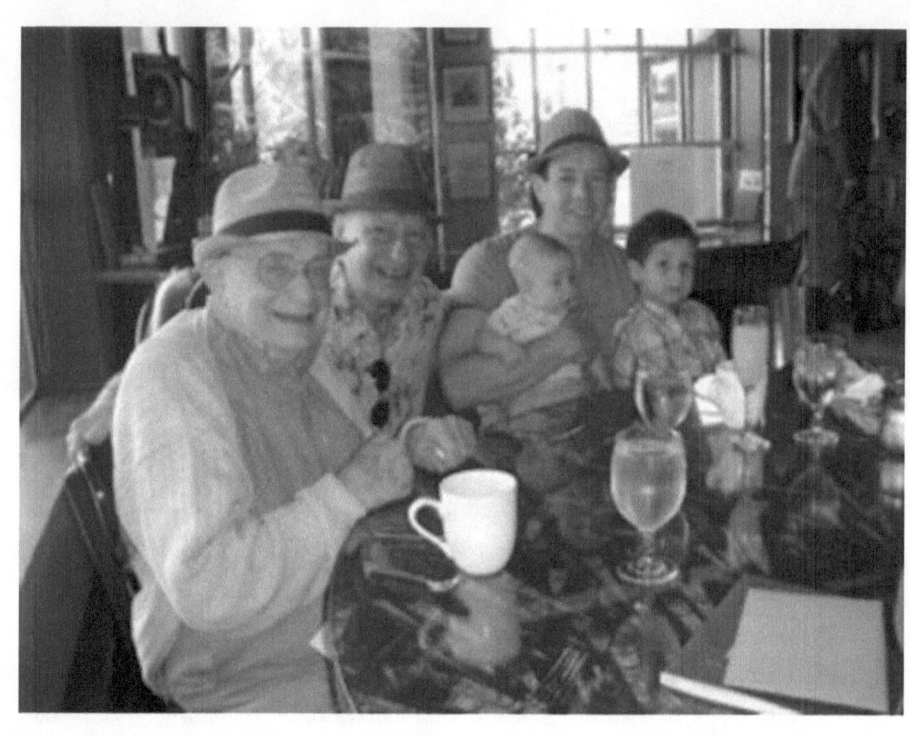

Chapter Ten

Life With Dad

True to his ornery nature, Dad is definitely keeping me busy and on my toes.

Early Summer 2011

I Don't Know What to Do

Dad has settled in and is not very happy. I'm getting calls on a regular basis:

Friday: "I'm out of bananas."
Tuesday: "I need you." "I need new shoes."
Wednesday: "Call the dentist." (Dad has dentures and only one tooth.)
Thursday: "Call my friends' children's father. I think he plays bridge."
Friday: "I need some things at Walgreen's."

There is always something. Unlike Mom, he can dress himself, shower himself, and feed himself. He just has trouble amusing himself. He is no longer using his computer, even when I walk him through the process. If I don't check his e-mail, nobody does.

The Routine

As in Mom's case, but with the active aid of my husband, we have developed a routine for Dad too. Every day he gets his Denver Post, which he reads while he eats breakfast in his apartment. Then he gets dressed and goes for a walk around the building. Often he stops at the first floor library to take out a new book. (He is known for reading the first three chapters and then returning the tome). Then he comes back to the room, makes himself lunch, watches a ball game or a golf tournament on ESPN, takes a nap and then either visits Mom or watches some more television or reads before he heads on down to pick up his mail before dinner at 5:30.

Frequently Dad invites us to join him at dinner. My husband will drive from work and meet me at Dad's and we'll visit a while at Dad's apartment and then all go down to dinner. Dad takes great pride in asking the waitress to bring wine to the table for all three of us, and he is very specific about what he wants me to bring him from the salad bar. A good day is when the dining room serves herring. Early in Dad's residence I meet one lady at Oak Tree who eats with her mother every night. I admire this, but with a mother, a husband, a son and daughter-in-law and two grandchildren, I know that plan won't work for me. I am forced to make my parents a little less dependent.

I have enrolled Dad in a dry-cleaning pick-up service, but I still have to get his shirts and slacks ready for the pick-up. Eventually he learns the routine, but it's always a struggle. Housekeeping cleans his apartment weekly but they keep switching the day. Yikes! Why can't they get their act together? I've tried to encourage Dad to just go downstairs while they clean but usually he wants to go out to lunch. I've taken him to Zaidy's, Racines's, Elizabeth's, 730. He likes them all once, but then he never wants to go back again. It's kind of like his reading habits. I think he's developing ADD at the ripe old age of 95.

Once a week I pick up his laundry and bring it back to do at our house. My husband thinks I should just pay the extra fee to have the residence do it, but I've paid extra for his apartment and I think I should make up for some of that amount by doing the laundry. It's not that hard.

I'm spending a lot of the time at the grocery store shopping for Dad. "Mir," he'll call and say breathlessly. "I'm out of bananas." Dad doesn't seem to be able to get organized enough to make a list. Actually, my husband has never been very good at this either.

Sometimes our children will go over with the grandkids to visit Dad. Mostly they see Dad up in the mountains on the weekends.

Passing the Time

Dad likes to find activities for me to do. Last week we went to the shoe store to buy him new walking shoes. That took a couple of hours. I haven't seen him wear the new shoes since we bought them.

The Takeover

Dad has requested that I take him to a tailor to have all his pants shortened. We go to our local tailor and the owners fall in love with Dad. He's such a cute man and they can't believe he's 95. He is pretty sprightly.

Dad has expressed an interest in me arranging a dinner with his friends' daughter's father-in-law. The father-in-law plays bridge and he is seeking him out as a prospect.

Tonight we dined with my father's friend's daughter, her husband and her father-in-law who is Dad's age and lives in Denver and is a bridge player. He is a little bit too aggressive and intellectual for Dad. The dinner was pleasant but Dad was very subdued. Maybe his expectations were too high.

There are many activities in Dad's building, but Dad shows little interest in any of them, Sandra, the dining director, continues to try and arrange company for Dad's meals. A couple of people have invited Dad to come to dinner with them. Jan, the activities director, has signed him up to attend a fall lunch.

"He didn't show up," Jan reported to me after the fall lunch occurred. She seems incredulous like this never happens. I don't know. I think it's not surprising. Jan relates best to the country club set that were the original occupants of Oak Tree. I don't think she has updated her approach since the demographics of the place began to change a decade ago, the time when she must have lost her enthusiasm for her job. Not soon after Dad arrives, she retires from her position.

Then there is Zelda Katz, age 102. "I placed a copy of the Jewish News in your father's mailbox," she tells me one day in the lobby. Wearing an attractive beige summer pants suit accessorized with large red stone earrings, she sits comfortably ensconced in a wing chair in the lobby where she frequently holds court. "When I came to Denver," she explains, "I knew nothing about the Jewish Community and the paper helped me learn about it." Zelda, who still walks without a cane or a walker, is a well-known fixture at Oak Tree. She can be seen at many of the lectures that take place during the week and she is an avid duplicate bridge player. Zelda is a bit much for Dad.

Today Dad asked me when his lease is up. "Three more months," I tell him.

Medical Matters

Dad has been complaining to the geriatrician about his urinary condition. The geriatrician seems to think his problems are normal for his age, but on my own I ask for a reference to go see a urologist just to check out Dad's current condition. The fact that he has had prostate cancer for over twenty years makes me think that occasionally it would be good for him to have a check-up.

I make an appointment to take Dad to see the urologist. He is very old and will retire the next month after Dad sees him. He's a gentle man and Dad likes him. He prescribes some medication to help ease Dad's urinary problems. Afterwards Dad and I go to lunch at Racine's, his restaurant of choice for the moment. We split a Reuben sandwich and Dad scarfs down the French fries.

Dad has told me that he is having trouble sleeping. I go to Walgreen's and buy an over the counter sleeping pill. I don't take many pills myself so it takes me quite a while to figure out which drug to select. When I mention Dad's sleeping issues to Dad's doctor during his regular visit to Dad, the doctor adds on a prescribed sleeping pill to Dad's medical regimen. Now Dad is taking two pills, more than he's ever taken before. He administers the pills himself. The sleeping pills seem to help. Each new prescription requires another trip to the pharmacy. There's no pharmacy service for residents in independent living.

Legal Matters

Dad has decided to remove Mom's name as the medical and financial power-of-attorney for him. He also wants all her mail sent to me instead of him. I am in the process of working with an attorney from my husband's office and with the insurance companies and Medicare to get all of this changed. More and more he is handing over all the financial matters to me. We are still having all of his mail sent to him, but he looks through it very quickly and then gives it to me. I have set up accounts on line for his bank and his investment company.

Father's Day

Today is Fathers' Day. My darling son has found a restaurant for us all to dine at and I have purchased "Mad Man" hats for all the men. I wrap them up in brightly colored tissue and place them in bags with golf balls and ties on them. We have a wonderful brunch (lots of eggs benedicts) and take a picture of the four generations of men.

Summer 2011

Weekends in the Mountains

We've been taking Dad to the mountains with us on the weekends. If we suggest that he might stay in Denver, he gets very agitated and we just say, all right, we'll all go.

The ritual is almost always the same. The day before we leave he'll call me up and ask me what he should pack. A few hours later he'll call me up and ask the same thing. On the day that I come and get him, he'll have packed his suitcase and will be waiting for me. Then we'll go down to the lobby and he'll tell the receptionist that he'll be away for the weekend. "I'm going to the country," he'll say.

In the mountains, he's content to just walk around the house and hang with us. Every morning he'll come out for breakfast and sing, "Oh, what a beautiful morning." My husband has graciously allocated his leather chair in his man cave to my father. That is a true sacrifice. I've never cooked so much in my life!!! It's easier for Dad if he doesn't have to go out to a restaurant since most of the restaurants require extensive walking and frequent stair climbing.

The summer symphony season has started in the mountains and we take Dad to the initial concert to hear the pianist who is also the music director for the festival. Mom and Dad had been avid symphony goers for years in Chicago. The logistics to get to the amphitheater are a bit tricky. We go very early so that we can drop Dad and I off on level ground. I worry about Dad making it through the concert, but he does fine. We take Dad to one more concert at the end of the summer. Otherwise we go to the concerts by ourselves and Dad is happy to stay by himself at the house.

My husband has decided to take Dad with him on a couple of business trips to the Western Slope. My father adores my husband and has always loved talking business with him. The first trip is to Grand Junction where he visits with my husband's partner and his wife whom he also adores. The second trip is to the casinos in Central City and Black Hawk where my husband meets with clients and Dad hangs in the gambling hall.

We went to see "The Help" last weekend. Dad hadn't been to a movie in twenty years. I think he enjoyed it.

No one wants to be with us since Papa Lennie came into our lives. Today Zeca (our grandson) went to a soccer game pizza lunch rather than come to lunch with my brother and his wife and my husband and Dad.

Dad is amazing in the high altitude. He has no trouble breathing or getting around. Several times Dad and I make the one hour and forty-five minute drive to the mountains separately from my husband because of my husband's work schedule. Dad is very content to look around at the mountains and always points out the arch that indicates the turn off to Central City, the place that he and my husband have visited together. He declares me a good driver, something that no one else in my family has done.

Finding Dad a Bridge Game

After a long frustrating search, I have found Dad a bridge game that he likes. Though the Oak Tree activities director tried to involve him with the bridge activities at his residence, he has never found a comfort zone. Some of the residents are pretty serious players and they only play duplicate bridge. Dad is more of a social bridge player.

I have done a thorough search around the Denver community for senior bridge games. I have contacted the Jewish Community Center and I think I've finally found something he might like. I am taking Dad this Wednesday. We'll see how it goes.

The elders at the Jewish Community Center have welcomed Dad into their bridge game with open arms!!! We went last Wednesday for the first time. Dad, now using Mom's old cane, dressed for the occasion. He wore his summer cap and favorite cotton cardigan sweater. We entered the hall where they play and he immediately found a partner. Her name is Barbara. She dresses beautifully, drives herself to the center, and uses a walker to get around. Dad says she "likes to take risks," but he says it with a chuckle like he doesn't mind.

It is now on my calendar to take Dad to the JCC on Wednesdays and to pick him up two hours later when the game is over. The JCC has a taxi service for seniors and Oak Tree also has a limo service but Dad prefers for me to drop him off and bring him back. Recently he invited me into the JCC hall because "everyone wants to meet you." They went on and on about how much they enjoy having Leonard join them. On some days I'll drop him off back at Oak Tree and then return to the JCC to pick up my grandkids who go to daycare on the same campus. My life is shrinking!!!!

Like Mom, Dad is also going through the same Medicare program for physical and occupational therapy. It's actually pretty helpful because the therapists are trying to teach him how to orient himself in the neighborhood. They walk with him, and they show him the best ways to navigate around his apartment and around the building. They have asked me to provide a calendar so he can begin to understand what he's doing each day, each week and each month. I help him write in his bridge days, the kids' birthdays, when we are going to the mountains and his doctors' appointments. He still gets confused. The doctor thinks he might be experiencing some dementia and adds another pill to exacerbate this possible condition.

September 2011

Mom and Dad's 70th anniversary is September 6th. I ignore the day, but my brother acknowledges it with a phone call. I'm sort of sorry I don't really have some festivity, not even a card. I think I am so exhausted that I'm just trying to get through the days. I'm happy that at least my brother acknowledges the event. We've had so many celebrations in the past, their 85th and 90th birthdays, their 90th and 95th birthdays, and their 65th anniversary. Later, I feel avoiding an acknowledgement was not such a great choice. I should have been more positive.

It's the Jewish New Year and we will be going up to the mountains to go to services. I've purchased a ticket for Dad as well. In preparation for the holidays I buy Dad a box of New Year's cards and tell him to send them to his Chicago friends. After a little bit of urging, he writes out a message that he copies onto each card that he sends. There are probably twenty cards. I address and mail them. Several of his close friends and relatives have already written him back or called him. Dad is delighted.

Taking Dad to services is as tricky as it was taking him to the concerts. We have to leave early because we need to get a parking space. That means we have to eat dinner out and near the chapel. We make it through the evening and day services for Rosh Hashanah and for Kol Nidre on Yom Kippur night, but we're just too pooped to do Yom Kippur day. I think, like the books Dad reads, he has tired of the services. My husband and I are fasting but Dad isn't. I run out to McDonald's to get him a breakfast before we head back to Denver. I haven't been to a McDonald's since my kids were young and it takes me a while to order. The clerk just shakes her head with wonderment at my laborious attempt to figure out my selection. I bring the breakfast back to our house and Dad, with great enthusiasm, chomps away. Then it's back to Denver where I make a Break the Fast dinner for the three of us and our children and grandchildren.

We are taking a hiatus from going to the mountains. We are remodeling the kitchen and have been told to stay away until it's ready for Thanksgiving.

We have changed our dinner ritual with Dad. My husband now brings a bottle of wine for us to share in the apartment before we all go downstairs to dine.

It's time for Dad to have a flu shot. He was unable to have Oak Tree administer the shot because they offered the service on Yom Kippur, so Dad and I go together the week afterwards to Walgreen's and park in the handicapped parking space and have another outing. Of course, we go out to lunch afterward.

We have returned to the urologist whose office is now occupied by a younger replacement for our original doctor who has retired and sold his practice to him. The new urologist thinks Dad's PSA level has soared and that the shots that he has not taken for some time should be resumed. I make the decision to do this. Later I worry that I did not make the right choice, but at the time, I was willing to go along with his advice.

October 2011

It's my birthday and I insist that Dad take me out to lunch. I choose a sort of gourmet cafe that is located next to a very popular bookstore. The place has good parking and it's a beautiful fall day. We have a lovely lunch and then go to the bookstore where I'm hoping Dad will browse around. He's always loved books. He doesn't browse but he is content to sit in one of the store's comfortable chairs while I look around for something to read. It's a good day.

My brother and his wife have come to visit Mom and Dad on their way down to Albuquerque where they are in the process of building a house. My husband and I are only too happy to pass the baton to them. They dine with Dad, walk with him, and watch golf with him. And, of course they see Mom as well. I have to say my brother has been very nice about checking in both by phone and with his presence.

Oak Tree has noted that Dad seems to be disoriented and has been making an effort to "integrate him into the community." We have a new executive director who personally involves himself in Dad's well being. He is young, enthusiastic, and has recently moved with his wife from Seattle to Denver. Originally from New Mexico, he seems open to new ideas, a lovely contrast to the staid, conventional approach by the former CEO who has just retired after twenty years at Oak Tree. It's kind of ironic that we are meeting with him once again. We actually met him in the elevator the day Dad moved into Oak Tree. He was pretending to be looking for housing for his parents and asked us lots of questions just to get a feel for whether or not he wanted to be the next CEO. While my brother is visiting, we have a family visit to his office with Dad where he and my brother talk at length about New Mexican cuisine. He suggests that I hire people from the caregiver department to amuse Dad and get him involved. I actually didn't realize how this department worked and felt, even though I knew it was in the financial interest of Oak Tree for me to use their services, that this was a very good avenue for me to take with Dad.

After the usual paperwork and bureaucracy kerfuffle, I hire caregivers to take Dad for walks twice a week and to a current events lecture every Tuesday. This is in addition to him going to bridge at the JCC every Wednesday, which he continues to love. Coupled with the World Series, I think he's in pretty good shape.

Despite all of these activities, Dad seems more and more down. I'll come and visit and he'll be sitting in his chair and he'll start to weep silently and put his hands up to his head. "I don't know what to do," he'll say. It makes me so sad to see him like this. His friends often check in with him and sometimes they just call me. His best friend has recently called me to report on a recent conversation he had with Dad. "You know, your father needs to practice all the things he learned from Dale Carnegie (the original self-help guru whose course Dad took when he was younger) about having a positive attitude." I am fond of saying things to Dad like, "I know this is hard, but think of all the things that are good. You have your health. You have darling grandchildren and great-grandchildren. You have great friends." This does not always work although when Dad's friends call him, they report back to me that he says he is doing very well and that we are keeping him busy. He never complains to them.

Someone has suggested that I ask the doctor to give Dad an anti-depressant. It has been common in my family to have bouts of depression. The doctor at first dismisses the need for any medication, but it seems to make him more cognizant of Dad's state and eventually he sends a professional out to do tests on Dad. A lengthy conversation several weeks later produces first an evaluation by the doctor's psychiatric nurse, then a report, and finally a prescription for some medication. The nurse also says that Dad has the onset of dementia and she prescribes a new medication for this condition. This entire process lasts a couple of months.

November 2011

Yikes! Bedbugs!

I have just received a call that my father's apartment has bedbugs! I am appalled and a bit humiliated by the whole thing. Oak Tree's maintenance director takes control. First he hires an exterminator and tells us that Dad needs to be out of the apartment for several hours. I bring Dad back to our house. The housekeeping staff launders his linens and his pillows and tells us everything will be back to normal by five o'clock. When we return, the linens are not there, the pillows are not there, and housekeeping is not there.

Lots of phone calls follow. Pillows are borrowed from a guest suite, the linens are returned and the bed is made up and, after a disquieting dinner where my husband joins us, we leave Dad at his somewhat rehabilitated apartment.

Our kitchen in the mountains is done just in time for Thanksgiving. My California cousin and his wife are joining us for the holiday and with my dad we will all be convening for the celebration and will be joined by our children and grandkids after Thanksgiving Day.

Thanksgiving

It's Saturday of Thanksgiving weekend and my husband has received a call from his sister in Chicago who informs him that his aunt has died and that the funeral will be on Monday. Simultaneously and unexpectedly his sister has been hospitalized with a sudden illness. My husband drives back from the mountains with my cousins and goes with them to the airport and flies to Chicago for his aunt's funeral and to see his sister. Soon after my husband returns from Chicago, his sister passes away. Our entire family flies in for the very sad funeral. Our son and daughter-in-law return immediately after the funeral and my husband and I stay on for four more days to be with my husband's family.

More Bedbugs!

We are back from Chicago and so are Dad's bedbugs. He has been asked to leave the apartment for several hours again, but not before the housekeeper shows me what those little guys look like. They are not pretty.

This time I take all of Dad's sweaters and pants to the cleaners to be fumigated and I take home all of the clothes in his bureau to wash in hot water. I also buy bedbug proof covers. I don't care about the cleaning bills or the time spent in the laundry room or the expense for the sheets. I just want it over.

Dad decides to stay downstairs in the lobby when the exterminator comes and promises not to go up to the room before the allocated time, but he doesn't keep his word. I leave him alone for a couple of hours when I get a call from the exterminator that Dad has returned to his apartment too soon and that the exterminator made him leave. Then I get a call from my disoriented father. I run over to Oak Tree where Dad is sitting in the lobby. I lose my temper for the only time since Dad has been with me. "Dad," I scream. "Why couldn't you wait?" He changes the subject. "I had lunch today with some very nice people." "Dad, how could you do this?" I rant.

It takes me a long time to get the bedbug image out of my mind, but so far we have not had another episode.

December 2011

Shopping for Zeca

We are going to be celebrating our grandson's fourth birthday on December 3rd and I tell Dad that he and I need to go shopping for a gift for Dad to give him. My shopping designation I decide will be the Super Target that is located nearby. Now equipped with a handicapped placard, I am able to park very close to the entrance.

My dad walks verrry slowly, and when we get inside, I say to him. "Let's look for a motorized cart."

Dad resists. "I'm not going to ride in one of those."

"Oh, yes you are," I decree emphatically.

When he realizes it operates just like the golf carts he used to drive when he was a younger lad, he is off and running. We go to the toy aisle, where he carefully selects a truck and then to the card aisle where he picks out the only card that says "Happy Birthday to my great grandson." I take home the truck and wrap it up and Dad presents it to his great grandson at the birthday dinner celebration.

Note to self: You're going to have to put your foot down with Dad. He's taking advantage of you.

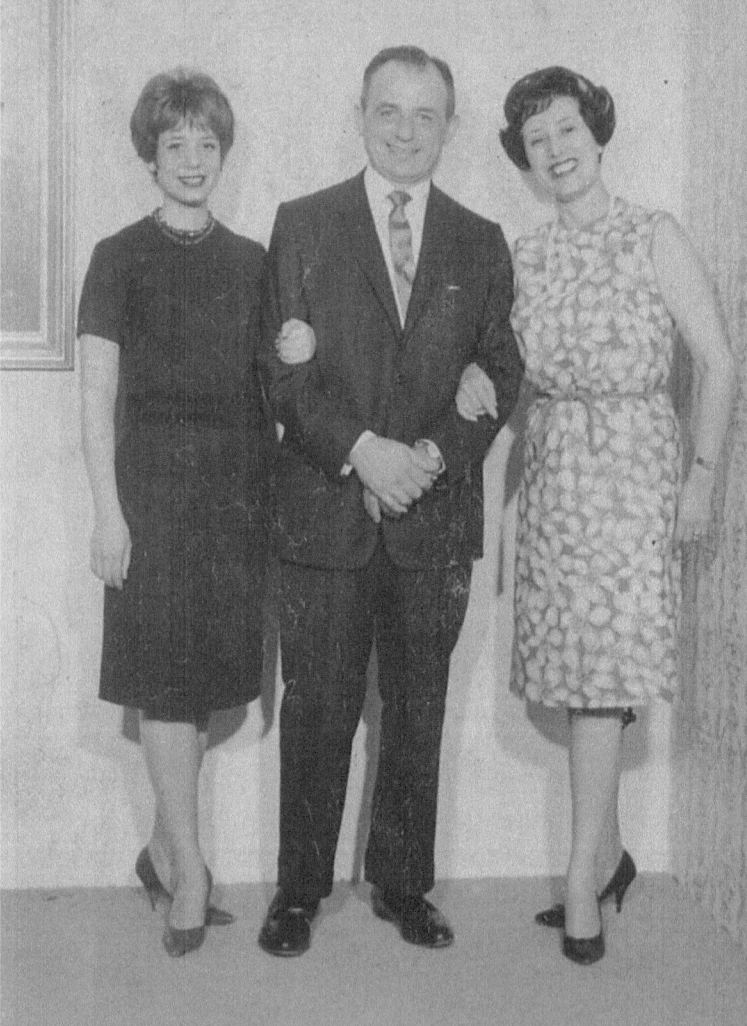

Chapter Eleven

Mimi's Daily Drill: Musings from Mimi's Blog and Journals

I am a tired cookie. I try to sleep whenever I can but then when I try to sleep, all I do is worry. This is not good.

June 2011

    CALENDAR:

        June 3rd
        Take Dad to the urologist

        June 13th
        Mom in ER with a gash in her head.

        June 14th
        My childhood girlfriend visits me and Mom and Dad

        June 24-27
        My brother and his family visit Mom and Dad on route to a family reunion.

        June 26th
        Take Dad to Vail for opening concert.

June 30th

My cousin Sadie comes to visit from California. She is warm and comforting and fun. She visits with Dad and then we go down to visit Mom. Their reunion is touching. I take a picture of them and wipe away the tears.

NOTES:

I am starting to return to a version of my old routine. I get up and have breakfast and watch Morning Joe and the Today Show. Then I go work out, two days a week with a trainer, four days a week running on the treadmill, and try to do yoga once a week. After I work out, I go to the grocery store or the cleaners if necessary. Then I come home and make phone calls and tend to chores like the laundry. Then I shower and make my way over to Oak Tree. It is only five or ten minutes from where we live. The challenge of parking around Oak Tree has become a hobby of mine. I have become quite adept at parallel parking on the side streets that surround the residence. Once a month the street sweepers come by and each street has a different schedule. If there are too many spaces on the street, it must be a street sweeping day and I restart my search. I don't want an expensive city parking ticket! The longer this takes, the longer I get to listen to Beethoven and Tchaikovsky on my favorite classical radio station.

My weight is going up and up. I run around but not at the gym. I get very hungry and crave comfort food.

I'm getting to know all of the people at Oak Tree who take care of both Mom and Dad. It's taken a while. The facility is going through a lot of organizational changes. The Executive Director who I worked with when placing Mom and Dad here has just retired after twenty years. A replacement for her has not yet been announced and there seems to be a constant revolving door with old staff members leaving and new ones coming in.

Normally I stop at Mom's first. This is after I call Dad whom I speak to several times a day and ask if he's going to come downstairs with me to see Mom.

I have started reading about eldercare. I have taken out one book that is categorized by subject matter and written by two public broadcasting experts and the other that is a personal story that I purchased over the Internet. The second is by a former New York Times sports reporter who took care of her mother during her last few years that her mother was alive and addresses all the complexities she dealt with. Even though she was only taking care of one parent and even though her mother had different problems, her struggle becomes my eldercare Bible. In many ways she is preparing me for what's to come.

The Takeover

I am knee deep in making sure that all the address changes for Mom and Dad have been updated. It's been quite a chore.

I have taken myself out for a leisurely lunch that included a very pleasant glass of wine.

The bills have started pouring in from Mom's stint in the ER. The first bills are from the hospital and the medical staff, known I quickly learn as "the providers." Their amounts are awfully scary. I'm not sure what part Medicare pays, what part Dad's supplementary insurance pays, and what part I owe. I'm on the phone with everyone, i.e. the insurance company, Medicare, the hospital. Half the time they're all missing some of the information, i.e. Mom's Social Security Number, her date of birth, her supplementary insurance, etc. etc.

I'm concerned about Mom's reparation checks that she has received from the German Consulate since the end of World War II. I ask Dad why we're not receiving them and he, of course, has no answer. I call the German Consulate in Denver, which refers me to the German Consulate in Los Angeles. Several conversations have now occurred and they have finally reinstated her status and have told me that monthly amounts will be forthcoming. It's not much but believe me, when you have two aging parents, every dollar counts.

Dad has asked me to change his medical and property powers of attorney designations. Dad wants to remove Mom from everything including the trust and to place my name on everything instead. I don't even know what half these words mean!!!!!!! We ask for someone in my husband's law office to help us sort this out. Then there are all kinds of signatures required including some from Mom. All must be notarized. Unbelievably, Mom actually provides some version of her signature. Now that the power of attorney has been legally changed, I must notify in writing every entity that needs to know. My learning curve on all of this has been lengthy. I have purchased a notebook and allocated a page for each entity. I keep redoing all of my notebook pages and have started a filing system. My Mom and Dad's paper work now takes up two drawers and a shelf. I am going out to buy file boxes to make the whole system clearer in my mind.

I am trying to simplify my life a bit. That's not easy. I'm trying to get Dad used to the idea of finding things to do on his own and I'm trying not to not check in on Mom daily.

Mom is actually more busy than Dad because where she lives the day is so structured. Dad is really left to his own resources to make a life for himself.

I have become an expert on incontinence. I know every venue that sells supplies and what types they carry.

It's now the end of June and we will be going to the mountains on the weekends for the music festival. I'm not sure that will be of interest to Dad.

July 2011

CALENDAR:

July 6th
Interview with a Medicare service to help me sort out all of the paperwork. Please, please let this work!

July 11th
Spend the morning at the Department of Motor Vehicles to get handicap placards and identification cards for Mom and Dad. The long wait is relaxing!

July 29th
Concert in the mountains with Dad

July 29-31
Our son and daughter-in-law in town from LA

NOTES:

I'm having a great time reading on my phone about my upcoming 50th high school reunion. I've reconnected with a bunch of people and am getting a great kick out of hearing everyone's memories. It's funny how high school seems so much more tolerable when you're nearing seventy and when it's your only relief from the constant tedium of life. The whole connection is a lovely counter to my increasing isolation from my friends.

Our son and daughter-in-law are visiting from LA. The whole family including Dad has journeyed up to the mountains for the weekend. On the Saturday before we have people over for dinner, the family goes for a hike. We leave Dad behind with the children's fifteen-year old dog. We return all exhilarated. As we walk into the house, Dad greets us with great consternation and guides us to piles of vomit in the hallway and bits of the filet mignons we were defrosting for dinner scattered throughout the kitchen and living room areas. It seems that the dog discovered the defrosting filet mignons on top of the kitchen counter. A bunch of cleanup follows before we pull together some sort of dinner for the family and our children's guests. On Sunday we all return to Denver where our son and daughter-in-law visit Mom. She is very happy to see them and thrilled with our son's gift, a Native American style painting he has drawn for her. She nods when we point out that the painting seems to have been influenced by the work of Fritz Scholder, a highly regarded Native American artist. I almost think she is coherent.

We've been regularly taking Dad with us to the mountains. At first we thought he would stay in Denver because when we go up we attend a lot of concerts and aren't always home a lot. But Dad looks so hurt when we don't include him that we just take him with and he sits at the house and watches baseball games. We leave on Friday and return on Monday morning. It's hard to take him out for dinner, so I've been doing a lot of cooking instead. The cooking needs to be soft because Dad has dentures and can't chew much.

August 2011

CALENDAR:

> August 3rd
> Elm Place BBQ
>
> August 9th
> Dad visits his urologist for a check-up
>
> August 10th
> Dad's bridge begins
>
> August 19th, 20th, and 21st
> Visit kids in LA
>
> August 26th
> Sabbath services with Mom and Dad at Oak Tree. Dad's cousin conducts the service.

NOTES:
Our dog has died. He had been acting strangely for quite a while and when I finally took him to the vet, they did some tests and told me he had terminal stomach cancer. If I wanted to spend thousands of dollars for chemotherapy, I could have extended his life a bit, but at eleven years, I thought he had had a good life. I decided to put him to sleep. I stayed with him until it was all over. It was very sad.

My husband and I are in LA visiting our younger son and his wife. We've just received a call from our son in Denver that Mom has fallen but she's all right. Our dear children have brought both grandkids to Oak Tree to visit Mom and Dad. They are terrific!

I have been trying to keep both Mom's and Dad's clothes in order and sort through them regularly. I do Dad's laundry once a week including his linens. I have tried to mark all of Mom's clothes with a Sharpie to reduce the constant loss of her clothes when Elm Place does her laundry.

I've had to take Dad back to the bank and put Mom's name back on the check register. Otherwise we can't cash her checks from Germany. Banker Chelsea was very deferential to Dad and he loved it.

Dad has decided that he no longer wants to receive any of Mom's mail and would I please change her address so that her mail is sent to me. I consult my now bulging notebook of places to notify and move on.

My solace is in my writing, which I try to squeeze in whenever I have a moment. In addition to my other blogs, I have started one called "Eldercare Diaries." It's very therapeutic.

September 2011

CALENDAR:

Back in the city until the end of November while the kitchen in the mountains is being remodeled.

> September 1st
> Missed Book Club
>
> September 2nd
> At the zoo with our grandson and his day care class because his mom couldn't make the date.
>
> September 9th
> Meet with Bath and Kitchen Planner
>
> September 12th
> Missed Girls' Lunch
>
> September 22nd
> Exterminator at house to assess the animal in the attic problem
>
> September 30th
> Baby sit for grandson while son and daughter-in-law are in San Francisco.

NOTES:
Taking a lot of naps.

Sometimes I think that being with grandchildren and being with my parents have a lot of similarities. We're working on potty training our grandson and we're trying to do the same with Mom. We dine with both the grandkids and with Dad. I have to admit the grandkids are a lot more fun.

I'm out of all makeup and toiletries. I keep running out of everything for myself and I never seem to find the time to catch up. Today I shopped for my winter wardrobe. In three hours, I purchased everything I think I will need. I knew I might never get another opportunity.

October 2011

CALENDAR:

> October 1st
> Jewish New Year in the mountains
>
> October 7th and 8th
> Yom Kippur in the mountains
>
> October 8th
> Break the Fast in Denver with Dad and our kids and grandchildren. I order out from Zaidy's!
>
> October 9th
> Contractor at house to address master bathroom leak problem.
>
> October 11
> My birthday. We visit Dad's new urologist and go out to lunch.
>
> October 17
> Senior Dental Services for Mom and Dad at Oak Tree.
>
> October 20th
> My brother and his wife are in town to visit Mom and Dad
>
> October 20th
> Meeting with the new Executive Director of Oak Tree on "integrating" Dad into the community. More paperwork and more money for extra services.

October 24th
Oak Tree Caregiving session for Dad. The caregiver and he go for a walk.

October 31
Halloween at Oak Tree. Pick up my grandson, Mr. Zebra, at his school and bring him over to Oak Tree to do a bit of trick or treating. Dad meets us at Mom's unit and watches as our darling grandson makes the rounds and visits Mom, who is not very impressed with Mr. Zebra. The residents except for one put candy into his pumpkin. Our grandson is very upset when one resident takes some of the candy out of his pumpkin instead!

NOTES:
I'm having a lot of trouble sleeping. I can't tell whether it's because I'm drinking a lot of wine or if it's because I'm so concerned about the welfare of my parents. I am constantly grappling with my decisions. Did I do the right thing by moving them out here? Was it right to place them in the residences where they're living? I take ten breaths where I count up to thirty. Sometimes this helps.

November 2011

CALENDAR:

November 3rd
Manicure and pedicure. It feels wonderful. Missed my book club.

November 4th, 5th and 6th
In AZ to visit my husband's sister and brother-in-law.

November 11
Dentist appointment for Mom

November 14th-26th
My cousin is in from LA for work. Staying with us in Denver

Thanksgiving
In mountains with cousins and Dad

Thanksgiving Friday
Children and grandchildren in mountains with us

Thanksgiving Saturday
Husband is called to Chicago for funeral of aunt. Also to visit his sister who has been hospitalized.

November 28
Mr. Pest Control for Dad's bedbugs

NOTES:

Fell and gashed my head in Oak Tree dining room on the night before leaving for Arizona. Was able to tape my head back together and avoid the ER! Amazing how no one in the dining room paid any attention to my fall!

It's a bittersweet visit to Arizona to see my husband's sister and terminally ill brother-in-law. More wheelchairs, but we have a good time anyway.

Can you believe Dad has bedbugs in his apartment??

I have been informed that unless Mom is declared incompetent by her doctor that her name will remain on the trust. So be it. We've been advised that most doctors have trouble declaring a patient incompetent and that we probably shouldn't even ask to have this done. I think I finally have the paper work in place for all the entities that need to know about the power of attorney conversion. Whew! That has taken months.

December 2011

CALENDAR:

December 1st
Visit Mom for the first time in a week. They think she has a urinary infection.

December 4th
My brother visits

December 9th
Mr. Pest Control back for a second application at Dad's place

December 10th
Mom's bell concert at Elm Place.

December 13th
Meet with the Medicare specialist. Not much help.

December 15th
Take car into shop. Miss holiday lunch with girlfriends

December 17th-20th
In Chicago for my husband's sister's sudden and very sad funeral. Children on duty for Mom and Dad in Denver after funeral.

December 25th
Christmas/Channukah/Birthday Brunch at our house

December 27th
Dad's birthday at Elway's

December 29th
Visit to two possible assisted living places for Dad

NOTES:
My car is in the shop again. It's been kind of a rough go for me carwise. First I decided to repair all the knicks in the car I drive around Denver. They did a complete paint job. Then I got two traffic tickets in a row for speeding. Then I stopped suddenly and someone crashed into our mountain car. Then I had to get that car fixed. Then Dad discovered that the paint was peeling on my Denver car that had just been repainted.

Dad's condition is worsening and I am looking into the possibility of moving him once more but this time into assisted living instead of independent living. Not only is he becoming less and less able to function, but also he seems very unhappy in the building. I'm thinking that maybe he would be better off with a less intense environment. The hustle and bustle of Oak Tree may be overkill. On the other hand, I say in my sleepless night fits, maybe change is not such a good idea.

Note to self: You need to reassess Dad's situation. I sometimes think that now that he is not needed as much, he seems to be falling apart. Do not even deal with the shoulda couldas. You made your choice. Now live with it and adapt.

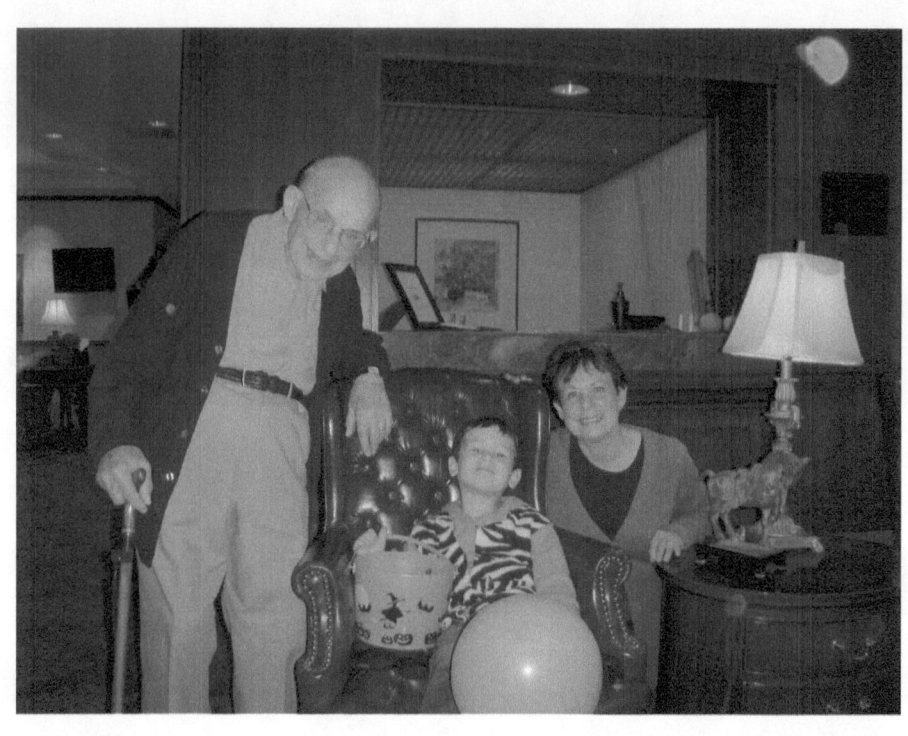

Chapter Twelve

Celebrating the Holidays

It's a bittersweet holiday. A lot of crying, a lot of laughing, a lot of work!

December 2011

December has been full of ups and downs. We have a very good time celebrating our grandson's fourth birthday, but this is followed by the sad news that my husband's sister has passed away suddenly after a very brief illness. The entire family attends the funeral in Chicago and then my husband and I stay on for a few days more.

When we return to Denver, we try to pull ourselves together to enjoy the holidays as much as we can.

The Bell Concert

Mom's unit has been practicing for a holiday bell concert since before Thanksgiving.

I try to ready Mom for the big celebration. I make sure her hair and nails are done and I plan out what she will wear.

Today is the day of the concert. I arrive early to dress Mom in the outfit I have selected for her, a red and green patchwork jacket. I haven't laid it out for the staff because the last time I laid out an outfit for an event, they never put on the specified outfit. When I arrive, Mom is already in the living room and she is wearing sweat pants and a turtleneck top. I bring in the patchwork jacket and clumsily get her to put it on. I am the only one who is dressing her parent as the bell lady directs everyone to their places. Why is it that I never seem to be on track? My husband and my dad arrive and Dad takes a seat next to Mom in the residents' semi-circle. My husband and I pull up chairs among the audience and graciously accept some eggnog and cookies that the staff is serving.

The director begins the concert. On cue each resident shakes his bell and lo and behold we realize we are listening to "Silent Night." After a few more carols, Mom seems to lose the rhythm and she starts to shake her bell out of turn. The director tries to be patient with her. Finally she says to her in the most polite manner that she can muster, "Liese, you did so well that we're going to take your bell and give it to someone else." Mom is fine with that. Apparently that's enough for her. Dad and my husband and I laugh and laugh at the whole event. It is festive and fun no matter how your parent performs.

The Channukah, Christmas and Mom and Dad Birthday Brunch

Though we are Jewish, traditionally our family has always celebrated Christmas in a big way. My mother's birthday is Christmas Day and my father's is two days after and Channukah is celebrated around the same time. In our house we have always celebrated Channukah and Christmas together and now that Mom and Dad are with us, I figure we'll celebrate their birthdays as well all on Christmas Day.

Part of the Pockross tradition of celebrating Channukah on Christmas Day is the purchase of eight gifts for each family member to represent each day of the Channukah lights. One of those gifts is the same for everyone. This year everyone is getting games. It takes me forever to find the gifts, a few of which are major and the rest sort of practical and then more time to wrap them all. Since our son and daughter-in-law live in LA, I get both of their eight gifts mailed out ahead of time. As holidays usually are, it is hectic.

I am very nervous about having Mom at the house. She hasn't come since Mothers' Day, and I won't let her come without a caregiver, mostly because I don't want to take her to the bathroom and I know I'll be busy with the food and the kids.

I drive myself crazy making arrangements for Mom. I hire a caregiver and make plans for transporting her on Christmas Day. I order the food including one birthday cake each for Mom and Dad, and of course I purchase a few presents for each of them as well.

The day goes perfectly. My husband and I go to Oak Tree together and I dress Mom with the caregiver's help. The caregiver and I wheel Mom downstairs where we meet my Dad and my husband, board my husband's SUV and make the ten minute journey to our house.

Both parents love the lox and bagels and their cakes and they love watching our grandson open all eight gifts for him plus the eight gifts for his brother who is way too young to understand the process.

Everyone else opens their gifts too and Mom and Dad share their individual birthday cakes with us all. It turns out to be a very fun day, I am relieved to say. Mom was just fine, slept through some of it, but we did it, and it was worth it.

Taking Dad Out for A Birthday Dinner

Two days later we take Dad to Elway's for dinner. Dad, a huge football fan, enjoys the restaurant connection to the famous Denver football player. Using his cane, he saunters to our booth where he revels in dining on French fried onion rings and a big thick, juicy steak regardless of how difficult it is for him to chew. All around us people look on in amazement as Dad, now 96, enjoys his meal.

New Year's Eve

We leave Dad in Denver for New Year's and go up to the mountains with our children and their friends. Dad signs up for the New Year's party at Oak Tree but he doesn't go. Being up in the mountains with our children, grandchildren and some friends of our children is relatively mellow after a very chaotic year. My husband and I go out for an early New Year's Eve dinner and we do some babysitting. It's always nice to be in the mountains. Mom and Dad are in Denver and manage well enough without us.

We welcome the New Year after a very sad ending. We mourn the loss of my husband's sister and we thank ourselves for all the good things that we have in our lives and that Mom and Dad are as good as possible under the circumstances.

We are all looking forward to a family celebration in Mexico for my husband's 70th birthday. This will occur only three weeks after the New Year. It will be the longest test for Mom and Dad to get along on their own.

What a year!! What will 2012 bring? We just keep moving on.

Note to self: Was that bell concert the funniest thing ever???? It felt good to laugh and I think Mom and Dad had a lot of fun. Those grandchildren are fun too! Now it's time to work on finding Dad a place in assisted living.

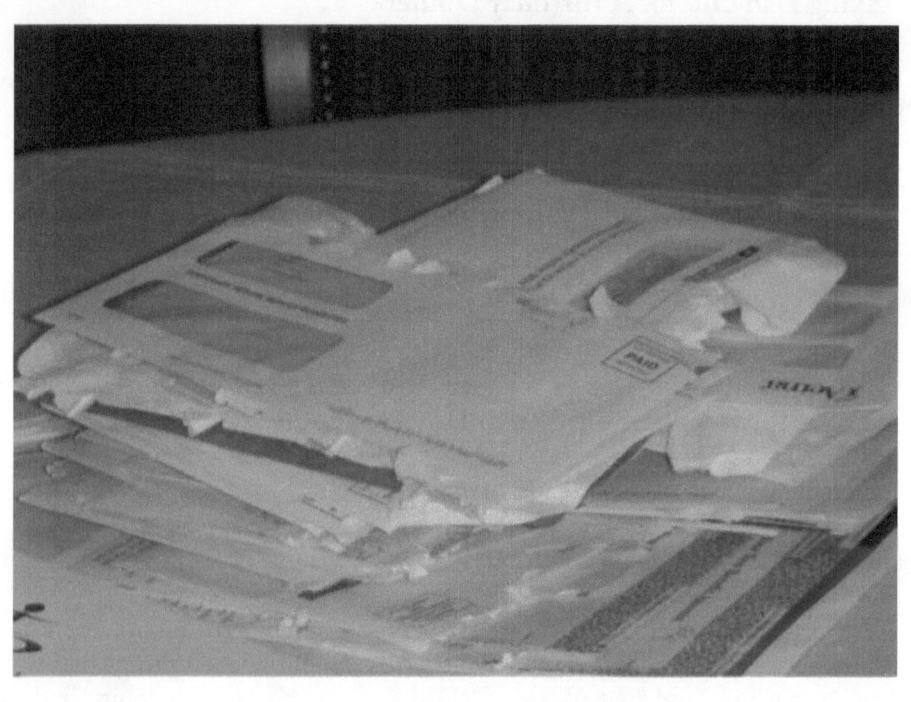

Chapter Thirteen

Going Downhill

Are you really going to Mexico for Keith's 70th and leaving your parents behind? What kind of nerve is that? I'm desperate. I know I'll pay for this.

Early January 2012

Mom has e-coli. The nurse's assistant assures me that this is a very common malady for older people.

Dad and I visit an assisted living unit at a different facility. Dad likes the place but not the room he would occupy. He decides to think about it.

The car is back in the body shop for a paint job redo.

Mom is back at the dentist.

One of my Denver cousin's has died. We attend the funeral to which I mistakenly wear a blazer instead of the suit jacket that matches the pants.

Getting Ready for Mexico

We are taking a family vacation to Mexico to celebrate my husband's 70th birthday. We will be gone for five days.

I have hired extra caregiving for Mom and Dad to help out when I'm gone. I have made up a sheet of informational material to hand out to all of the staff at both Mom's and Dad's living quarters and I have arranged for transportation for Dad so he will not miss his weekly bridge game. I have told all the administrative staff as well that we will be in Mexico and I have made sure that everyone has a copy of our plans.

Mexican Mishaps

January 12th
All eight of us have arrived in Mexico and are enjoying the sea and the sun

January 13th
Our daughter-in-law has been called back to Denver from Mexico to take care of a burst pipe in their home and to move their family temporarily into our Denver home.

Our son and grandchildren remain in Mexico with my husband and I and our other son and daughter-in-law

January 14th
8:00 am: Our daughter-in-law has moved their belongings into our Denver home. She calls to report that their fifteen year old dog has passed away during the transition. Lots of tears.

10:00 am: Dad calls from an ambulance where he is on his way to the Emergency Room. His condition is diagnosed by the staff as a Urinary Tract Infection. At the ER, the doctor inserts a catheter into Dad and returns him to Oak Tree where from Mexico I hire round the clock caregivers from Oak Tree's caregiving unit. We are not due to return to Denver for four more days and we cannot cancel our reservations.

5:00 pm: I have received another call from Dad. He has returned to the ER for the insertion of a larger catheter. This time he is accompanied by our hired caregiver who also returns to Oak Tree with him. The caregivers work on shifts. One stays with him at the ER and then when he returns to Oak Tree another one takes over.

There is no guarantee that the same caregivers will be assigned to Dad each day and night. Dad, of course, is very upset.

January 16th
Our son and his children are back in Denver and with our daughter-in-law now living at our house. They check in on Dad periodically to make sure he is comfortable.

January 18th
We have returned from Mexico and I've just gone to see Dad. He was sitting in his recliner with the catheter sticking out and the caregiver was sitting next to him. My heart goes out to him. He's just so disoriented and depressed.

The children and grandchildren are now living with us until their house can be repaired. Though it's an adjustment, they are a great diversion from the intensity of caring for my parents.

Nursing Dad

I have been nursing Dad back to what I hope will soon be his regular self, but things are not going well. For the first week after Dad's return from the ER, I continue to keep the caregivers on a rotating basis. Thursday I take Dad to the urologist to remove the catheter. Acknowledging my father's wishes, I reduce the amount of caregiver hours to three times a day for two hours at mealtime rather than around the clock.

It is the first day of the revised schedule and I go to see Dad. He is in the bathroom hardly clothed, the living room is in shambles and there is garbage all over the place. The caregiver helplessly is standing by. Only at my request does she stay and complete my orders to clean up. It is past her contracted hours.

I try to figure out what to do next. My first thought is to rehire the caregivers from Oak Tree around the clock. I have left several messages first with the caregiving department and then with both the administrative assistant and the reception desk since the caregiving department has not returned my calls. I have told each of them my problem: Dad is by himself except at meals and when he is alone, he is not able to take care of himself. Please get someone to take care of him as soon as possible. Knowing that the dinner caregiver will be arriving soon after Dad's afternoon nap, I go home to rest and wait for the phone call from someone at Oak Tree and to mull over my current situation and come up with some options. I don't think I'm capable of doing the caregiving myself. I'm lucky enough that I can hire people. Aside from moving in with Dad, which I don't want to do, I just don't see how I can help him and perform all the other obligations to Mom and to my husband, house and children.

Help!

The phone rings and Cindy answers. I think it's Cindy, the administrative assistant of Oak Tree. I am so grateful that someone finally has returned my call. I tell her the situation and ask her what I should do and she suggests respite care. I'm somewhat familiar with the term. It means sending your loved one to a facility that can temporarily help with extra care for your parent. "That sounds great," I say. When we continue our conversation regarding the alternative, I realize that I am talking to Cindy, a marketing director at Horizon, a different facility, not Cindy at Oak Tree where Dad lives. Oh well, I'm desperate and if it means moving Dad, what choice do I have? Respite care sounds to me like the answer. It's the only way Dad is going to get constant attention and as far as I know Oak Tree does not offer this service and who would be around to tell me if they did anyway?????

Note to self: Try to find some experts to help you deal with Dad. Enough is enough. For the life of me I can't figure out why Oak Tree doesn't provide any support. That's just how it is. You need to pick up the slack.

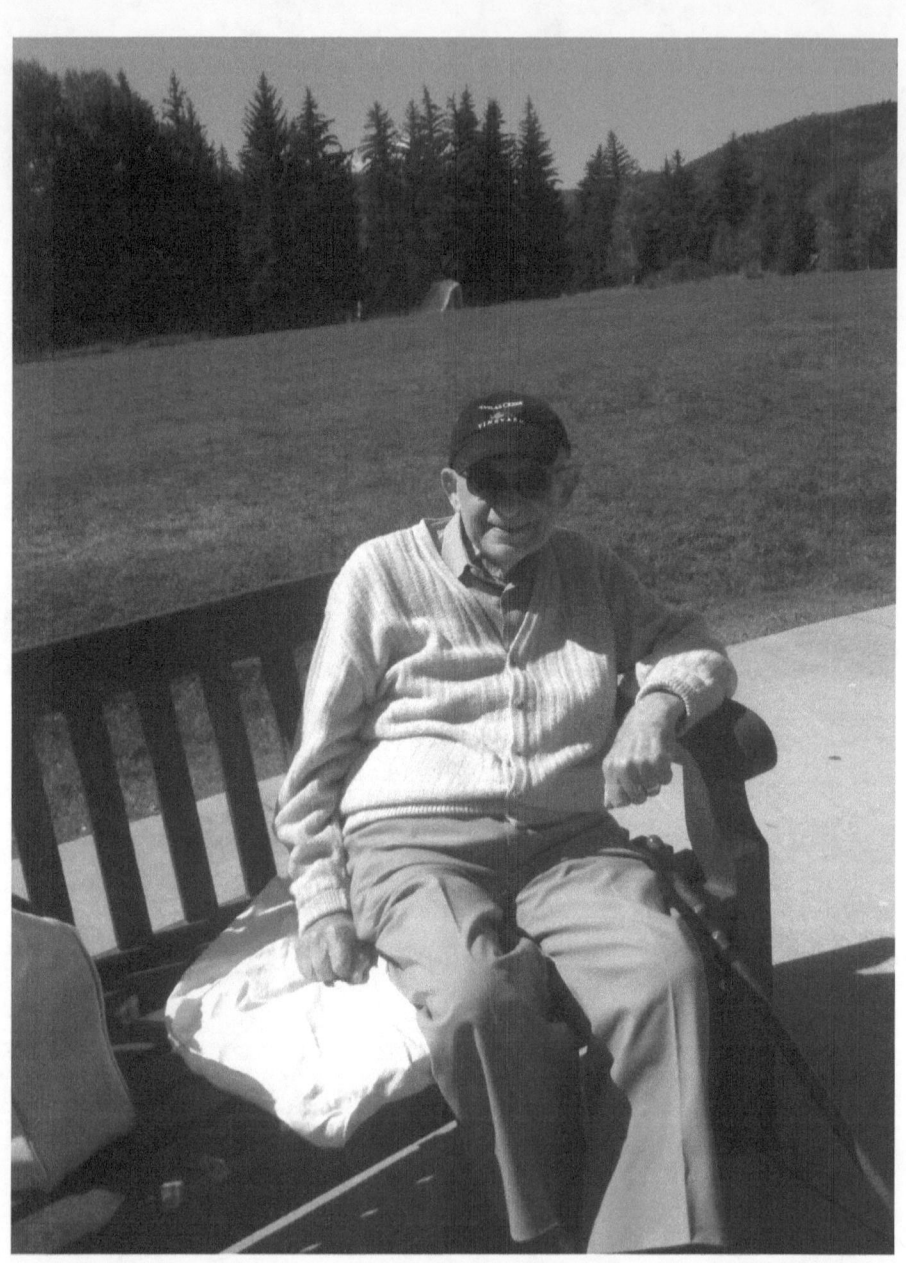

Chapter Fourteen

Dad Goes to Respite Care

Now I'm really in a bind. I've got one parent in respite care, one parent in a dementia unit who could get kicked out any time. I need help.

January 2012

The Transfer

The next day after I have contracted for Dad to be sent to respite care at Horizon, I make the ten-minute drive over to meet the director, the head nurse and Cindy, the marketing person who made the initial contact. I fill out a lot of forms and then figure out how to get a copy of Dad's tuberculosis test to them. He cannot be admitted without this form. After our meeting, the director sends a nurse and the head of resident services to meet with Dad at Oak Tree and to examine him. Both members are interested and gentle with Dad, and Dad finds this comforting.

As my husband and I pack Dad up, put on his coat and help him into a wheelchair, I'm still smoldering from the lack of response I've received from Oak Tree. It's Friday evening around five o'clock. I lock up Dad's apartment and wheel a very confused Dad downstairs and into the lobby where some sort of reception is taking place with all the Oak Tree staff present. I see Diane Denton, the Oak Tree caregiving director who has ignored all of my phone calls and I give her a very dirty look.

"Where were you when I needed you?" I blurt out.

She answers, "It was my birthday yesterday." How's that for dedication?

Of all the people I've worked with so far, she has reminded me most of everything that I don't like about the eldercare world. She is self-absorbed and pious. It's all about her. She needs some classes in empathy and she needs to know what a professional is, i.e. someone who does not bring her own personal life into the care of both the resident and the resident's loved ones. I don't care if my parents are living in a facility run by a large corporation. They can do a better job of training even if they aren't warm and fuzzy in their delivery.

Though I'm very angry, I am more concerned about getting Dad to Horizon, which I'm hoping will be more sensitive to Dad's needs. We navigate through the crowd and out the door, transfer Dad to the car and head the mile or so away to Dad's temporary new home.

We wheel Dad through the doors into the lobby and there are several people who welcome us. The receptionist is there. Cindy, the marketing lady who talked me into moving Dad is there. She's waited around on a Friday night to greet us. And one of the nurses who examined Dad in the morning is also around to say hi. The whole atmosphere is so much more inviting than Oak Tree.

We wheel him down the hall of the "Hollywood" wing that is flanked by posters bearing photos of James Stewart, Grace Kelly and other famous movie stars to his new quarters. His room is on the second floor.

"Are you OK, Dad?" I ask. "How does it feel?"

"Weird," he says in his new weak voice.

Horizon has provided him with a bed, a chair and a television in his one room "apartment." The room also has a bathroom and a refrigerator and a closet. I've brought along a suitcase for overnight with the intention of bringing the rest of his clothes over the next day. Right now we just want to get him situated.

We place the limited supply of clothes that we have packed in the closet and drawers and ask that his dinner be sent to his room.

It takes a while to provide the necessary information to the staff regarding Dad's current medical needs.

It's been a long day and a long week and we are all exhausted.

After Dad has settled down and we've met the night crew, my husband and I leave Dad with his cell phone to deal on his own through the night.

I'm not really that worried about leaving Dad. I think Horizon will watch over him. The assisted living unit seems to be more hands on than independent living.

Nevertheless, bright and early the next morning, I'm back at Horizon to check in on Dad.

The New Horizon Routine

The first few days that Dad is in AL have been intense as we try to acclimate Dad to his new surroundings and his new routines. It's definitely a relief to know that he is being monitored more carefully, that he is being bathed and dressed and fed on a regular basis and that someone dispenses his medications. Since Dad is only here temporarily, I have to supply all of his medications, which are then handed over to the staff and administered to him on a regular basis. They know me well at Rite-Aid. AL toilets him regularly and makes sure he remains dry and comfortable.

Horizon's staff has its issues as well. New caregivers don't dump the garbage, use up all his laundry without replacing it, forget to take away his breakfast tray, and frequently don't come up to visit him, but it's better than IL at Oak Tree where no one knew what Dad was doing and it's better than trying to oversee rotating caregivers who do very little. It's less costly too.

Dad's doctor from Oak Tree continues to see him at Horizon. For the most part, the caregivers who are assigned to Dad's floor are attentive and helpful. In addition Dad is receiving occupational and physical therapy as a follow-up to his ER visits. I have finally learned to be a bit wiser and have hired an independent home health service to do the therapy. Dad's doctor has recommended them and there is no comparison between the lackadaisical treatment offered by home health at Oak Tree and the treatment he is receiving from this independent company. Unlike at Oak Tree, they call and tell me when they're coming to see Dad and then after they've been there, they either write a follow-up report or call and let me know how it went.

On the recommendation of the occupational therapist, we have purchased a new walker for Dad so that he can walk up and down the long corridors and go downstairs to dine with the other residents.

Horizon is much more intimate than Oak Tree. The residents sit at the same table everyday, and on a rotating basis there are activities in the downstairs living room. Dad never attends. It's cold outside so it's not possible to take Dad for walks. Besides it's not really a very pretty neighborhood in which to walk.

Dad's table in the dining room is the "men's table." Mostly they all sit in silence and eat their soup, salad, entree and dessert. One man is very ill with cancer and getting ready for a difficult chemotherapy treatment. At first I try to make conversation at the table and then, when that proves to be unrewarding, I just talk to Dad occasionally. It's not a very joyous environment. Oak Tree is much more upbeat, but then most of the residents in their dining room are in IL, not AL. There's a big difference.

Sakina, one of the caregivers at Horizon, has taken a liking to Dad and has turned out to be a great help in watching over him. A hardworking woman who has immigrated from North Africa, she is always there for Dad and never lets him falter.

Our children bring their kids occasionally to cheer up Dad and indeed that brings a smile to his face. We are lucky to have them here.

Dividing My Time

I am now running back and forth daily between Dad at Horizon and Mom at Oak Tree.

Amazingly, Mom seems to be in good spirits and relatively maintenance free while Dad is going through his rough times. I visit her when I can and she seems content. I'm not sure she has any idea what is going on with Dad. I do try to explain to her in simple terms that Dad is not feeling well.

Dad at this point seems to be the bigger problem since we are all getting adjusted to new circumstances, a new level of living and new bureaucratic issues. I am checking in on him daily and sometimes more. I am working with his physical and occupational therapists to try and get him back in shape. I try to encourage him to take walks with his new walker. Most of the time he demurs. Instead we put him in a wheelchair when he consents to go downstairs to meals, which isn't very often. He can no longer concentrate on anything. He no longer reads and he doesn't even express any interest in watching his sports programs except occasionally.

At this point I still have aspersions of going back to a somewhat normal existence. Even though I need to divide my time with Mom and Dad at two different residences, I still attempt to take time out for other activities.

We reschedule some plans to entertain some people up in the mountains that we had to cancel after our return from Mexico when Dad became ill. I am reluctant to leave Dad but I also feel that it would be good for me to have some down time. I am too tired to cook so we go to our favorite gourmet store and select some ready-made dinner to bring up to the mountains and serve to our guests. My phone is by my side the entire time that we are away, and I return to Denver the next day immediately after the dinner.

Dad has lost his hearing aid in the ER room. I am now investigating how to replace it. I have asked a hearing expert to visit Dad at Horizon.

I have been in contact with the new CEO at Oak Tree. He has been kind enough to take a personal interest in our situation and to make an effort to see if we can work out something where Dad would move back to Oak Tree and move to the assisted living unit. I think he realizes how difficult their company has made our lives since Dad's ER visit and he is being very helpful and accommodating in trying to move Dad back to Oak Tree. I would certainly welcome having both parents in the same place rather than doing the dance between residences that I currently need to do.

For some reason, our house has no heat. I'm waiting for our heating service to arrive. We can't have grandbabies in the house with no heat!

Our shower door in Denver has shattered and we are showering in shards of glass. I call our kitchen and bath planner and she brings in her troops. The workmen are in and out for a week.

Note to self: The operational style at Horizon is smaller and more intimate. I'm still trying to decide if their style is any better or worse than Oak Tree's.

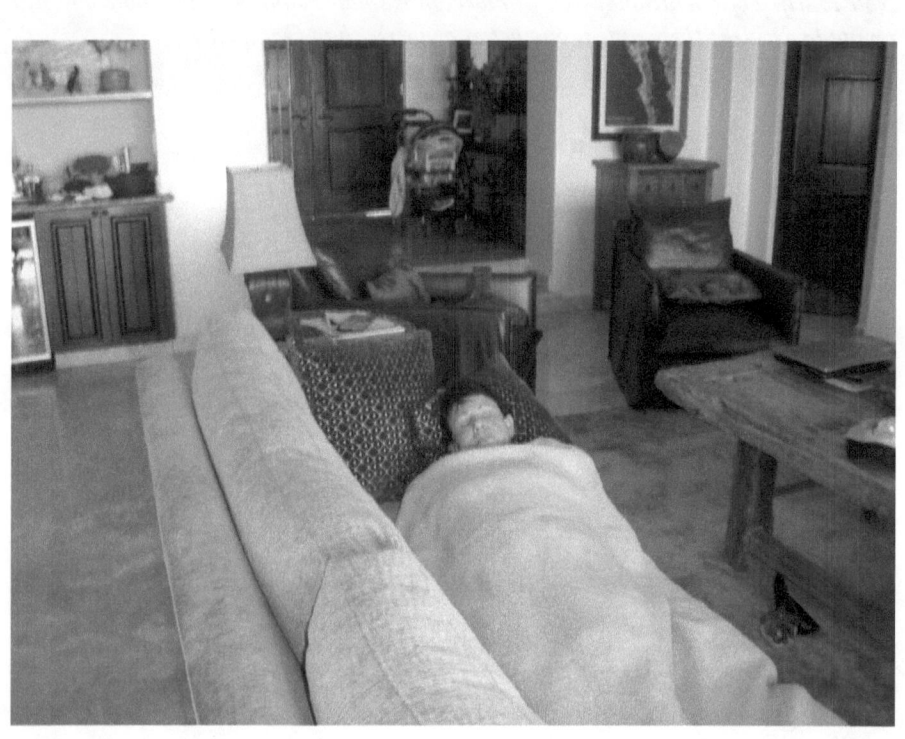

Chapter Fifteen

Hiring a Care Manager

A care manager sounds like the perfect antidote to my problems. Now if I can just find one.

Early February 2012

Now that I have two parents with increasing difficulties living at two different venues, I am trying to figure out the next move. Should Dad return to assisted living at Oak Tree or should he move permanently to Horizon? What am I going to do with Mom if I continue to get calls about her being aggressive and Oak Tree declares that she can no longer stay at Elm Place? Decisions will have to be made quickly and I don't think I have the correct resources in my toolbox to navigate. I also need some relief. Taking care of two parents is emotionally and physically draining and I have other obligations, i.e. taking care of grandchildren, overseeing two homes one of which is being remodeled, and trying to take some time out to do my personal chores and relax a little.

As I do each time I get frustrated, I take to the internet and I revisit the books I have purchased for assistance.

After rereading parts of "A Bittersweet Season," in which the author relates her decision to hire a geriatric care manager, I decide that maybe I need one too. I know I need some counseling of some sort. I have already given up everything except exercise and am having trouble sleeping and functioning in general. Though I don't have a full time job like the author and her brother did, I do have two parents with double the demands of just taking care of one.

The way I understand it, a geriatric care manager works with you on any level you need to provide the appropriate care for the ailing loved one. In Denver, which has very few such agencies, rather than providing any specific analysis of what the patient currently needs, their work is usually done in tandem with caregiver service, which produces more income for their company than care management. I am really looking for advice more than I am looking for caregiving. I am also looking for someone to occasionally take over responsibility for my parents when I leave the city to visit our home in the mountains, which is two hours away. I also want an agency that can provide a caregiver if my husband and I want to travel. For some unknown reason at this point I still think I can do this.

Once again I have returned to the Internet referral service that helped me when I was originally seeking housing in Denver for my parents. On my own I have also looked up companies that list themselves as geriatric care managers. There is a professional association of care managers and I refer to them as well. There really isn't much to choose from—it's a relatively new field—but I decide to give it a try anyway.

The Interviews

I interview three possible candidates.

The first one I visit is a very professional service. They are members of the National Association of Care Managers. Their staff are all gerontologists or people with advanced social work degrees. They patiently listen to my sob story for quite a while and explain to me how their system works. They need to fully evaluate each parent before they can make any recommendations. Then they will prescribe some sort of regimen. I'm thinking to myself, "this will take months. I'll be in the insane asylum by then." I leave somewhat dissatisfied but not sure why. I think they service the elite in the community and have a very exclusive clientele and, though they are caring and intelligent, I'm not sure they are up to date on what's currently available. Ironically, months later I see one of their staff taking care of a resident in my father's AL unit.

My second interview is with a company, which primarily provides caregivers and just kind of gives advice. I have met with the owner and the head social worker of the company and they seem very earnest and dedicated. Both have advance degrees in gerontology. They aren't sure whether they can help me with my needs.

The third contact I make is with a man and a woman, Sonia and Liam, who own a relatively new agency that "does everything" without any regimen or routine or contract. The interview is over the phone. All of this should have been a signal to me that the company was not quite working professionally. My perception was that they were shooting from the hip. Neither was a social worker. They started the company because they both were caregivers to relatives for many years. For some reason, this seemed like the sort of thing that I needed right now. Besides, they were both from Chicago, a comfort zone I always like. I hire them immediately. This decision turns out to be a disaster but not right away. Although they were recommended by the Denver senior care agency, in the long run, their abilities to perform in a professional manner fell short.

On Duty With the Geriatric Care Manager

Sonia has started making the rounds with me. She is rotund, wears a beret at all times and looks like a bossy lady in a children's cartoon. She visits Mom at Elm Place and immediately alienates the staff by offering suggestions for improvement and snooping around at Mom's charts. The theory of this very aggressive person is that you have to make your voice known and that if you don't speak up, you'll get left behind.

Soon after she is hired, Sonia arranges a meeting to discuss Dad's and Mom's status and to introduce herself to the staff at Oak Tree including the head nurse and the executive director. We are trying to figure out whether to send Dad back to Oak Tree or have him permanently remain at Horizon. The staff at Oak Tree is more than willing to meet with her since they were so negligent after Dad went to the ER while I was in Mexico. The Oak Tree staff all assures us that Mom and Dad will be well cared for at Oak Tree and that Dad is definitely a candidate for assisted living and will do very well there. I'm somewhat skeptical about their promises. I recall how Mom got kicked out of assisted living at the last minute while she was on the wait list for the Oak Tree dementia unit when Mom and Dad first moved to Denver.

I have begun meeting with the bathroom planner to help remodel all four of our bathrooms in our mountain house.

My brother has taken pity on me and made the airplane trip from Chicago to spell me. I don't remember ever being so happy to see him. It's good to have him around while we are trying to figure out what to do with Dad. While he's here, he visits Dad at respite care and we also make an appointment at Oak Tree with Amber, the marketing director to see what's available in assisted living there. Amber is very sweet and very concerned.

She has just lost her Dad to Alzheimer's disease and she knows just how difficult this aging process can be.

After Sonia meets with the Oak Tree staff, she does not really weigh in one way or another as to what is best for Dad. It doesn't matter though because my husband and my brother are insistent that Dad move back to Oak Tree and take up residence in assisted living. Their choice is more for my sake than for Dad's. At least this way, I will no longer feel like a ping pong ball. I eventually give in but not without a few reservations. The people at Horizon have really been trying to get Dad to stay with them. Of course they would. They need the residents and the staff works hard to encourage me to keep Dad with them.

In the course of trying to make a decision someone suggests that I investigate the Ombudsman's reports that the local area on aging must publish for each assisted living residence. It turns out that Oak Tree has none, and Horizon has one. I confront Horizon's head nurse and executive director about the incident and though they offer a defense, the fact that someone has accused them is enough to convince me finally that Oak Tree will likely take care of Dad as well as Horizon. I am also swayed by the fact that in the three weeks that Dad has been at Horizon, several staff members have left including the Executive Director. The staff turnaround in all these places seems to be frequent, no matter which choice one makes.

My husband and I then meet with Amber at Oak Tree and begin the process to move Dad back. I am so tired at this point that Amber and my husband figure out the tentative furniture arrangements. I then take home the packet of papers that are needed to be filled out before Dad can be transferred and once more await the approval of Helga, the head nurse who initially turned Mom down. I pray that this will not happen to Dad. The proposed transition will take place on February 21st after our son and daughter-in-law's visit to Denver from LA.

Our older son is in Orlando. We are on baby-sitting relief duty for four days.

Our younger son and daughter-in-law are in from LA to ski. With a new geriatric care manager in place and Mom and Dad entrenched in living quarters that are currently suitable to their needs, we try again to establish a new pattern of normality. We all go up to the mountains.

Mom Goes Back to the ER

Early Sunday morning my cell phone, now permanently attached to my whereabouts, rings loudly. It's Selena from Elm Place.

"We had to send your mom to the ER," she says. "She was quite violent last night and we couldn't calm her down." Elm Place's policy is that if a resident is violent, she must be sent to the ER.

I call my new geriatric care manager and ask if she can go over to the ER and take care of Mom until I arrive. She says she'll go right over.

I pack up quickly and make the hour and 45 minute drive back from the mountains. Luckily the weather cooperates.

Mom is lying in her ER bed, relaxed and enjoying all the attention. Sonia, as usual wearing her beret, sits next to her in a chair and is mopping Mom's brow and making sure she is comfortable. The staff is miffed. She seems just fine.

Shortly after, the ER releases her but not before another mound of forms is filled out. I'm smarter this time about how Mom will be transported back to Elm Place. I'm aware that if I order an ambulance, Medicare will not pay the seven hundred dollar plus bill.

It takes another 45 minutes after the papers are filled out before the logistics of dressing Mom, placing her in the wheel chair and making room for me to pull up the car to the ER entrance can be performed. Sonia is inside with Mom while I am waiting outside for a nearby parking space to open up. As I wait, I observe another patient in a gurney who, with his family, is waiting outside in the cold air for an ambulance to take him away. We both wait and wait and wait. Such is the nature of the ER world.

We return Mom to her unit and again hire a caregiver for the next 24 hours until she is stabilized. But I am very concerned about Mom. Something is bothering her or she wouldn't be acting up like this. There are several theories. She may be in pain. The doctor or his aide will come by and check this out within the next day or so. They have put her on more sedatives and some pain relievers. Sonia thinks she might be having psychological problems and suggests a therapist. I mention this theory to Helga, Oak Tree's head nurse who cynically laughs off the idea. She doesn't care much for Sonia anyway.

My own belief is that Mom's upset over the death of her best friend. My brother has relayed this information to her when he last visited. I'd been too afraid to tell her, but my brother is always more upfront. He was also the one to acknowledge Mom and Dad's 70th anniversary when I chose to overlook it. My theory is why upset the applecart, but my brother always prefers to face the facts. She might also be upset because of Dad. That only comes to me a year later!

On Sunday our son and daughter-in-law pay a visit to Mom at Elm Place and Dad at Horizon and then head on back to LA.

Our older son is in London this week and we are again on baby-sitting duty.

I just received another call about Mom being agitated. This time they do not send her to the ER.

Note to self: You are going to have to figure out alternatives for Mom if she continues to be aggressive. Elm Place cannot keep her if she cannot be controlled. Sonia is short on suggestions.

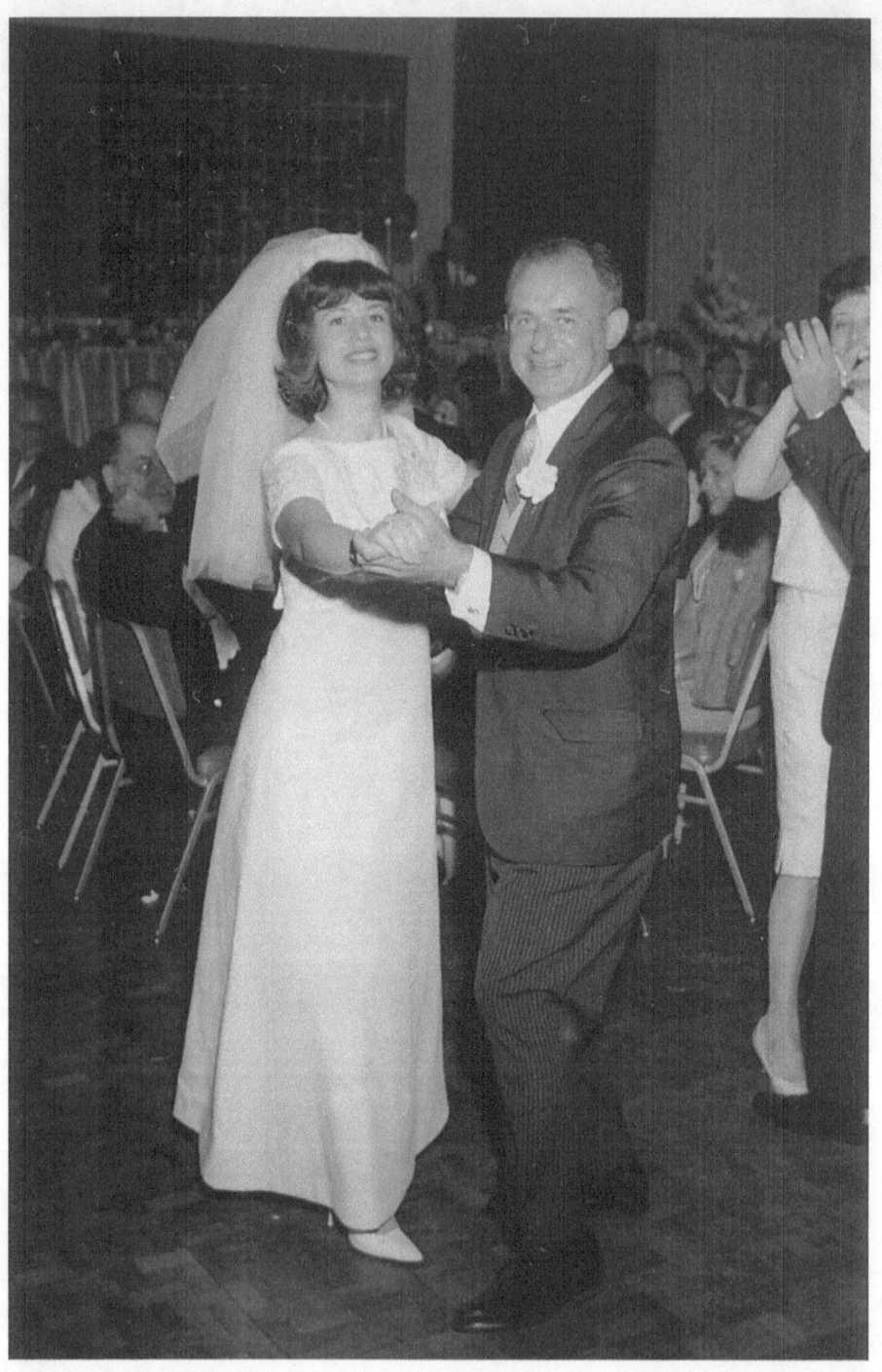

Chapter Sixteen

Dad Moves to Assisted Living

Having my parents one floor apart is very good exercise if you take the stairs rather than the elevator.

We Move Dad Back to Oak Tree

Again we have hired Ed, our "resident mover" to help us out with moving Dad down from the sixteen floor of Oak Tree's independent living quarters to the third floor of their assisted living units. After he moves the furniture and clothes and necessities that we have determined can be used in Dad's smaller quarters and he places the furniture in the configuration that Amber and my husband have defined, he loads the remaining furniture and boxes onto his truck and brings them to our house where he transports them down to our already packed basement.

On Monday, late in the afternoon, my husband and I pack up Dad, put him in his newly purchased wheelchair, transfer him to the car and drive him back to Oak Tree. He has been in respite care for a month. The staff at Horizon is very gracious as they bid farewell to Dad. Everyone who is around at Oak Tree pleasantly greets Dad as he returns.

The new apartment is nice and airy. Ironically Dad has a view over the patio where Mom's unit is situated. The apartment has just a few utensils, glasses and dishes, a television, a bed, a couch, and Dad's favorite easy chair that we had purchased when he first moved to Denver. A small baker's rack, a coffee table and two chairs and a table fit in the tiny kitchen area, and there's a place for his dresser drawer as well. Again, my husband hangs the familiar pictures and I place his *National Geographic*, his *Newsweek* and a few family pictures around to warm up the place. On the day before he moves back, I go out and buy a blooming plant and place it in his apartment for his homecoming.

Sonia suggests that we have a caregiver from her company to help ease Dad into his new surroundings on the third floor. The caregiver comes for three days. I decide to treat myself to a massage. It feels great.

Sonia comes to visit Dad and together we actually wheel Dad down to visit Mom after he arrives back at Oak Tree. They hold hands, Mom in her chair near her walker and Dad in his wheelchair. It's a scene I still vividly recall.

Now Mom and Dad are one floor apart from one another. Instead of taking the elevator which is vey slow, I take the back stairs. Sometimes I find myself going up when I should be going down or going down when I should be going up. A little bit extra exercise is not so bad. I guess I'm a bit disoriented. At this point, even if the paper work is overbearing, and it is, I'm very glad they are back in the same building. It takes several weeks before Dad is on a scheduled personalized living plan. Until then I have to be the one to continually remind the staff of what they are supposed to be doing.

Dad now eats in the assisted living dining room and is mostly confined to a wheelchair.

Now I, and often my husband, go with Dad to dinner each night to help him get used to eating in his new dining room. The atmosphere is kind of morose here. It's a temporary setup until a more expansive dining room is remodeled. Everyone's needs are greater. There are more wheelchairs, more walkers lined up in the hallway. The staff works very hard to accommodate everyone, but service is not quick. After all, where do these people need to be???? I like Dad's table. There is a silent but very independent gentleman who knows how to take care of himself. There is Helen who used to come into my art gallery many years ago. She's well past 90 and, unlike my dad, extremely vocal about her needs. "Can someone get me some water?" "I would like some dessert now." Etc., etc. We quickly learn that because of the crowded facilities, it's difficult to join Dad.

Not too long after his move, Dad's journeys to the dining room wane and he starts to spend more time in his own apartment.

Mid-February

Everyday paperwork for Dad's transition goes on and on.

I have finished the process of converting the medical and property power of attorney to myself for Dad. I have now changed the Power of Attorney two times, first to remove Mom and to substitute me, then to remove Dad and make me the sole medical and property power of attorney.

I have fired the Medicare service. It seems when they put in a claim for Mom's walker, they used Dad's social security number and now that we have put in a claim for a walker for Dad, the claim has been rejected. You gotta love these people.

I have hired an accountant to take care of Dad's taxes. We meet initially and then he asks me to pull together a lot of information, all the caregiver records, and the bills for Mom in her dementia unit. It's been a bit time consuming.

Dad's doctor has ordered oxygen for Dad. He seems to be having more and more breathing problems and is talking in a whisper.

Our daughter-in-law is in London and we are on extra baby-sitting duties.

Our son is in Las Vegas. More baby-sitting.

The New Drill

It is nice to have Dad in assisted living rather than having him fend for himself. At least occasionally caregivers show up to take care of him. Mostly that's confined to meals and dressing and occasional toileting. Of course, I want more even though I know the ratio of staff to patients is not one to one.

So far Mom has held up surprisingly well through the whole thing. I tell her about Dad, but I'm never sure how much of that she absorbs. I visit her in between my Dad visits. I abbreviate everything. "Dad is sick," I tell her.

I have started reading "Tuesdays with Morrie," a book from the nineties by Mitch Albom, the sportswriter who became a companion to a dying man. I want some support and the book is comforting to me. I recommend it to Helga, the insensitive head nurse at Oak Tree and give her my copy after I've finished.

Helga, the head nurse, is an enigma to me. She's the one who rejected Mom from Elm Place initially and who is now considering placing Mom and Dad in Oak Tree's hospice program if they do not show signs of improving. As head nurse, she oversees the assisted living and dementia units at Oak Tree. Her office is separate from both units. Occasionally I see her making the rounds, but as I observe her position more and more, I realize that she is overburdened with responsibilities. Along with hiring and supervising all medical and caregiving personnel, she is also in charge of making up the contracts for both the residents and all the services that provide the departments with products such as pharmaceutical and medical supplies. This requires a lot of coordination that is often done through endless meetings.

She never smiles. I attribute this to the extreme pressures of the job as well as to the fact that as a second wife in a blended marriage she is also caring for six children. (One day she shares this information with me). Not only that, but every time there is any emergency or abnormality in each of these units, it is her responsibility. That means she is always on call. I actually have some sympathy for her, but I keep thinking that if she would read "Tuesdays with Morrie," she might learn to have some emotions.

I've written an op-ed to the Denver Post on the symphony. It's a perk that it has been published.

Wow! Have I been giving money to the political campaign! Way too much, but it makes me feel good.

Note to self: I am beginning to understand that, though I value routines, in eldercare there are lots of interruptions and that's just the way it is. Just make your life as simple as possible.

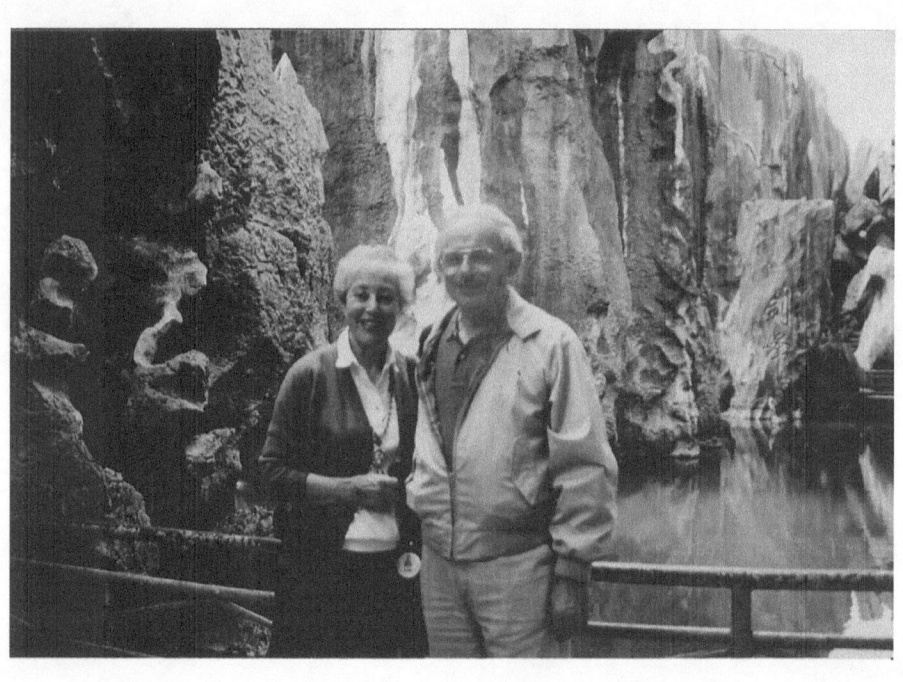

Chapter Seventeen

Hospice for All

Hospice sounds ominous, but you know, it also sounds like a very humane way to live with the inevitable.

Late February

Since Mom's return from the ER, there have been an increasing number of disturbing incidents. Today I got a call that she shook the television off the stand. Several times in the past few days, the Elm Place nurse assistant has informed me that she's scratched her caregivers. She is spitting up her pills. Her appetite is diminishing. She's weaving in and out of being stable. Her behavior is becoming more and more erratic. One day I'll get a call about some incident. The next day she'll be back in the living room sitting in her favorite chair with her feet up on her walker. I've stopped e-mailing my brother about her quick demise. The doctor has increased her sedative dosage.

Dr. Higby and I have already entered into a discussion about placing Mom in Oak Tree's hospice program, but until now he has been reluctant to recommend Mom for the program. To his credit, Dr. Higby, who I would describe as pretty much a naturopath, has been consistent in his using quality of life as the basis for his decisions about Mom. In the past he has reduced her medications so that she does not sleep all day and he does not actively work at making Mom "better." He just tries to keep her going. Until this point, she has been functioning quite nicely.

After this round of incidents, though, Dr. Higby finally concedes that Mom's condition is deteriorating and he recommends to Oak Tree's nurse that Mom be considered a candidate for hospice, a program that is just beginning at Oak Tree and is being supervised by Dr. Higby. Helga quickly (unlike in the past) approves of the move and again the paperwork begins.

The Concept of Hospice

Initially my understanding of the concept of hospice was that it was a program administered either in the home or at a separate facility with the mission of making a patient comfortable as he is getting ready to die. I was not aware that Medicare will pay for a hospice program for an individual who is not expected to improve and that as long as they "qualify" for the program, they can continue being treated without being discharged from the service. I was aware that there were a few residents in Mom's unit who were in hospice and had been for long periods of time. At one point when Mom first moved into Elm Place, one of the caregivers had actually suggested that Mom might be a possible candidate for such a program.

Though the definition of hospice varies by country and region, essentially the hospice program is concerned with providing a patient who is not expected to live very much longer with both medical and emotional support. Rather than doing everything possible to nurse the patient back to good health, hospice's interest is in accepting the reality that the patient is not likely to improve and to concern itself with doing everything possible to make the patient comfortable. I'm not sure where the distinction lies, but I did see many advantages to enrolling Mom in the program.

Ironically, it turned out that Dr. Higby had recently been appointed to oversee the new hospice program for Oak Tree. The new organization was being designed as a prototype to eventually service all local Meadowlands (the parent company of Oak Tree) facilities so it was really just in the experimental stage. Having used other Oak Tree supplementary organizations like Caregiver Services and their home health unit, the thought of contracting any other Meadowlands' associated group made me more than leary. I consulted my geriatric care manager. She suggested the names of some other hospice centers as possible alternatives, but I really think, because of what Sonia's company did, she preferred to think that caregiving was a better alternative.

Of course, I briefly consulted my books and the Internet. I learned that there are almost as many types of hospice programs as there are home health programs and oxygen supply companies!!! The eldercare world is a flourishing business.

Dr. Higby explained to me how the hospice program works. Under his supervision, a team of six people would attend to Mom. A director would determine her needs. Three nurses would monitor her medical situation and bathe and groom her, and a social worker and a spiritual counselor would provide emotional support for both Mom and me and my family. In addition to explaining how the program worked, Dr. Higby also provided me with reading material to learn more about the philosophy and implementation of the hospice program. He had done quite a bit of lecturing and writing about the subject.

It does not take long for me to decide to go with Dr. Higby's new hospice program. Although I have had difficulties with Oak Tree's other services, I have faith in Dr. Higby and am hoping that perhaps his department will be more competent than the others have been.

Mom Enters Hospice

On Saturday, February 23rd I meet Sloan, the director of Oak Tree's hospice program and begin the process to enroll Mom. After our lengthy conference and more paper work, she accompanies me down to meet Dad and then we wheel Dad down to Elm Place so that she can meet Mom as well. It is a touching scene as Mom and Dad face each other in wheelchairs while Sloan and I chat. It will be the last time they will see each other.

On Monday, the hospice wheels begin to turn. A new hospital bed is ordered for Mom's room and a mat for the floor is placed next to the bed in case she falls out of bed. AL units are not allowed to confine their patients in any way so a bar to hold her in is not acceptable.

In the meantime, oxygen is ordered for Mom to be used only as needed.

Once again, we call our mover Ed to take some of Mom's furniture to our house to make room for her hospital bed.

I meet the social worker and the spiritual counselor and the rotating nurses. Everyone is warm and consoling and empathetic. In a way, just talking about the situation seems to help things a bit. The hospice team organizes a meeting with the staff at Oak Tree for the next week and asks me to attend.

The doctor has decided to take Mom off all of her medications and increase her pain medications and her sedatives. He carefully explains the situation to me and indicates that the prognosis for her to get better is not hopeful, but Mom is so miserable and uncomfortable, I cannot see any reason to mix all those medications inside of her with questionable results. Though I have my moments of feeling guilty for not doing more to keep her going, most of the time I believe I am making the right choice. I do not tell Dad about hospice and I don't tell Mom either.

Dad Enters Hospice

It's the next week, and the doctor has decided to recommend hospice for Dad as well. Dad has also taken a turn for the worse. He has stopped eating regularly. He is becoming less and less functional.

"I thought after he returned from Horizon, he might rally," Dr. Higby states, "but it just doesn't seem to be happening."

Again it is time to fill out a paper trail, to call the movers to take away Dad's bed and put it in our basement and to have a new hospital bed placed in Dad's unit. Oxygen is also delivered in case Dad needs it, which turns out to be the case almost immediately after it is delivered. There is a lot of confusion over which oxygen unit should be delivered to which parent and it takes a week or so before we get it straightened out. A different oxygen service was used for Dad before he entered hospice, so the original equipment had to be returned and new equipment from the new provider brought in. Then the portable unit went to Mom who did not need the portable unit. We are using the portable unit for Dad now when we take him on walks and outings.

Hospice at Work

Mom and Dad are both now in hospital beds with mats laid on the floor below their beds in case they fall. They both have oxygen tanks in their rooms, and though Dad is always on oxygen, Mom has yet to use hers. Mom is on morphine and is no longer on any medications since she spits them out whenever they are offered. Her heart rate has dipped to new lows and she weaves in and out of awareness. Dad is on Ritalin to help him combat his sinking depression.

I have had to learn how to refill the portable oxygen unit and transfer the stationery unit to the portable one when we take Dad for outings. For a person who chose to be a teacher rather than a nurse because I am unmechanical and tend to be queasy this is a huge accomplishment!

I don't tell Dad about hospice except to say that we have some new people taking care of him who will make him more comfortable. I rather doubt he would understand if I told him the whole truth. I sort of regret a bit of this later. I know my brother would have been more upfront. I was of the opinion that Dad really didn't want or need to know more than the basics. At this point he has become completely reliant on my decisions.

I'm grateful that more people are watching out for him and still hopeful that he can work himself out of this new status.

The team meets both parents on a regular basis or if I call them up about a problem, they appear upon request. I hope it's comforting to Mom and Dad. It definitely is to me.

The hospice conference for Mom takes place the week after Dad enters hospice. On hand for the meeting are the hospice staff, the Oak Tree head nurse, and myself. Sonia, the geriatric care manager, is in absentia. She doesn't respond to my phone calls and she hasn't shown up as I requested.

"This is painful," I say to myself as I view the team seated around the table in Oak Tree's conference room and get ready for their questions.

The meeting is presided over by Rosemary, the vivacious and enthusiastic social worker but everyone participates. They want to know the whole family dynamic which is complicated to say the least. It is not fun to revisit all the painful parts of your family's history, i.e. Mom's emigration to America from Germany in 1938 and the subsequent extermination of her family during the Holocaust, the combative relationship that Mom and Dad have always had over their children and their lifestyle, the ups and downs of their financial situation and more importantly how each of them copes. Mom is a fighter. Dad is a downer. Mom adores her son and always criticizes her daughter and disapproves of her. Dad adores his daughter and has little respect for his son and his family. Despite all of the history, it's not a bad life when you sum it up. Why do they need to know all this? I'm a dishrag when it's all over. I'm definitely ready for a glass of wine.

The Hospice team has quite a bit of advice for me, which is reinforced in their calls and meetings either by chance or by appointment.

"There's no need for you to be around all the time," Rosemary, the social worker, avers. "The likelihood of you being present at the right moment is next to impossible. Take time for yourself. Separate yourself from the situation so that when you're with your parents, you can be at your best."

I have not been sleeping well. Mostly I worry that I'm making the right choices. When I think something needs another opinion, I call my brother, but really he just tells me to do whatever I think is best. The good thing is that we, who have all our lives sparred with one another, seem to be in agreement for the most part. At each stage I have told him the situation and chosen not to proceed without his approval.

Knowing that we would soon be facing the inevitable with both Mom and Dad, I have begun to make some preliminary preparations for their burials. With the help of my daughter-in-law's sister-in-law I have purchased two cemetery plots at the cemetery set aside for members of our former temple. Though the cost is more for non-members and the most expensive of all the three Jewish cemeteries, I still am comfortable with my choice. Mom and Dad have cemetery plots in Chicago, but I feel that it's better for them to be buried in Denver near where both my brother and I can visit their graves. We have already decided to have a memorial for both of them in Chicago after they have both passed away.

I think I'm living hour by hour now, going through the motions of checking in on each parent daily without looking backwards or forwards. I know that in both my mother and father's units, a lot of people are around them. Thank goodness the care seems to be good.

My husband and I try to keep both of them as comfortable as we can. The hospice staff does as well. The social worker and the spiritual counselor both drop in to see Dad periodically. A hospice volunteer who is the mother of the spiritual counselor comes to see Dad on Wednesdays just to spell me now and again. I think it's good too for Dad to have someone other than me to talk to.

Our son is in Las Vegas, and we are on baby-sitting duty again.

My husband is on a golf junket with one of his client friends. I think he just wants to get out of the house of chaos. We love the kids but it's high energy all the time. I find it soothing. It takes my mind off everything else to feed or bathe my grandkids or to read them a story.

My son and his wife are finally moving out of our house with their kids. Their house has been repaired after the pipes burst during our Mexico stay. My daughter-in-law has just returned from a ten-day business trip to London and they are moving their things back this weekend. We have been instructed to stay away while the transition takes place. That's very thoughtful of them. In between taking care of my parents, for the last ten days while my daughter-in-law was away, we've been spelling our son by helping take care of the kids. Our son will leave for Paris after the move has taken place. He visits with Mom before he leaves.

Note to self: Read up on Hospice. Read Dr. Higby's article about hospice as well. The more you know, the better you will be able to cope. Realize that neither one of your parents is likely to get better.

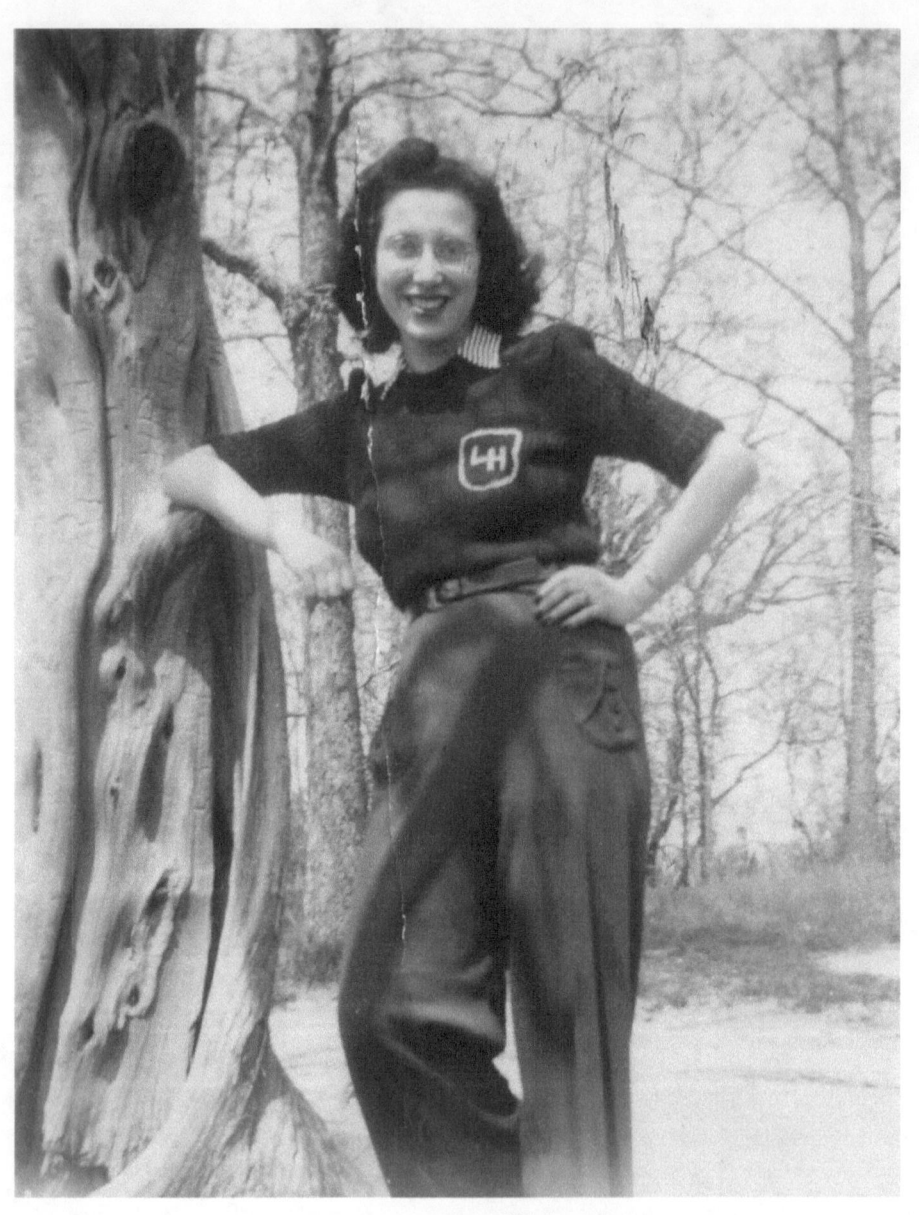

Chapter Eighteen

We Lose Mom

I think Mom passed "in style."

March 2012

Nearing The End

Mom has once more taken another turn for the worse. She is very weak because she can no longer take her pills. She is more and more confined to her bed. The staff has been instructed to turn her every few hours so she will not get bedsores. One day she'll be down, but the next day she'll be back out having some soup in the dining room and sitting up in the living room for a while.

I have brought a boom box and installed it in Mom's room. I've turned it to classical music, which Mom has always loved. I'm hoping this will soothe her and make her less uncomfortable.

Each day I visit Dad and spend some time with him before going down the flight of stairs to see Mom.

I tell the children not to bring the grandkids. They are sweet because they think that will cheer Mom up but Mom is not alert enough to know what's happening. They do go see Dad and he loves that. We're all on duty taking care of them both.

The Elm Place caregivers have stopped dressing Mom. They cover her with a nightgown and then with blankets. I'm not happy with this and go out to Target to find some sort of lounge outfit for Mom to wear that's easy to get in and out of and that I think will make her feel better. I bring it back and model it for her. She opens her eyes and looks at me for the last time I later realize. In my mind I have told myself that she approves. The staff then dresses her in the outfit. I'm feeling like I've done all I can. I sit with her for intervals and touch her and make sure she's comfortable. She's got her music and she's now dressed in her new lounging clothes. I say good night and, after visiting with Dad, I head on home for another restless night of sleep.

At 5:30 the next morning I get a call from the nurse. They think Mom's time is near. I put on my workout clothes and hurry on over to Oak Tree. I'm prepared to stay vigil. My daughter-in-law, fresh back from London, calls around 9:00 and asks if she can come over and see Mom. I say of course. She comes over and sits in a chair next to Mom and strokes her gently and in a very soft voice tells Mom about all her happy memories of being with Mom, of their times visiting in San Francisco, of her and my son's courtship and marriage. She's there for a good fifteen minutes before we leave to go see Dad upstairs.

When my daughter-in-law and I return to Elm Place, the staff informs us that Mom has just passed away peacefully. My daughter-in-law and I hug each other. Then I call my husband who comes over immediately and then we go see Dad. I call my daughter-in-law's sister-in-law who works for the local Jewish funeral home. I tell her that Mom has passed away and she quickly takes over the arrangements for moving Mom's body to the funeral home. Then we go see Dad. From Dad's room, I call my brother and hand the phone to Dad.

Dad is still trying to make peace with himself about his relationship with Mom, even at 96.

"It's all right, Dad," I say when we hang up the phone with my brother. "You were a good husband. Look, you were married for 70 years and you raised two great children." He cries silently as I have sadly seen him do so often these last few months. I think he is sad at the ending but I also think he is so sad himself that it makes it difficult for him to really focus on Mom's passing. His life is really caving in on him at this point. Together we call the rabbi at Mom and Dad's temple in Chicago and the rabbi talks to Dad. This helps.

Planning the Funeral

We will have several days before the funeral can take place. Mom has passed away on a Monday and our one son can't get home from Paris until Thursday night and our other son can't get out of LA until Friday morning.

The Takeover

It takes a while to locate a rabbi. We are not affiliated with a synagogue in Denver, and we think it's too far for our rabbi in the mountains to travel in to Denver to conduct the service. The funeral home helps us locate a rabbi and we schedule a meeting with him for Wednesday morning. My brother arrives on Tuesday from Chicago and he and I meet with the funeral counselor. By Wednesday the rest of his family has arrived and settled into our house where they will remain until after the funeral. The timing for this is really ironic since our children and grandchildren just moved out of our house the week prior.

The funeral home meeting is surreal. Though I've watched scenes of picking out caskets and meeting the funeral directors in movies, to be doing this for my parent is a new experience. My husband and I have already buried his parents and two of his closest cousins as well as his sister who recently passed away, but with the exception of one of his cousins, this is the first time that we've had a hands-on experience. Having a funeral counselor walk one through the process is a godsend. As instructed, I bring clothes for Mom to wear; my brother composes an obituary, which the counselor processes for both the local Denver paper and one in Chicago. Together we are led into a room of caskets and without too much trouble, we both agree on a simple oak one. The funeral counselor then proceeds to handle the burial details at the cemetery as well. We make arrangements for a time and for two limousines to pick up our family for the ceremony.

On Wednesday, we gather at the rabbi's office to tell him about Mom. I have asked my Dad if there is anything he wants to say about Mom. He wants to remind the rabbi about how very difficult it was for Mom when her family was killed in Germany after she had come to America.

The rabbi is kind and thoughtful with his questions. We are a lively group even without my two sons being present. It is not very difficult for him to get a picture of the person who was my mother.

It is agreed that the two oldest grandchildren will speak, as will my brother and myself. Years ago my mother had told me that she didn't want me to speak at her funeral, but I have finally in my old age learned that I can respectfully disagree with her, so I elect to say just a few words.

I hire the same caregiver from our care manager's company that has spent time before with Dad. I ready Dad's clothes and prepare Dad as best as I can for the day of the funeral.

In the meantime I cater food and order flowers for after the funeral and hire a server. We have decided on graveside services and have discouraged out of town relatives and friends from attending the funeral so we don't think too many people will be present for the service nor for the dinner afterward.

The Funeral

The day of the funeral arrives. Both sons are back in Denver. Since our house is full, our younger son is picked up by our older son and stays with him until he returns to LA.

I get dressed quickly and my husband and I head over to Oak Tree early. Even though we have hired the caregiver and told those in AL to get him ready, I have a feeling that things will not go smoothly. I am not surprised when we arrive and find Dad in the bathroom with terrible stomach problems. He is weak and unable to stand at all. When I arrive he collapses in front of my husband and me and I have to lift him up into his wheelchair. There is discussion with the caregiver on whether or not he can even attend the funeral. She thinks he shouldn't go, but I am determined that he can get there. Somehow we get him dressed, attach the portable oxygen tank, place him in the wheelchair and wheel him downstairs and out to the car. We drive back to the house where the limousines and the remainder of the family are waiting and drive the short distance to the cemetery. It is a very warm March day. I think Dad is comfortable once he gets in the limousine and is surrounded by his family.

We gather at the cemetery plot. To help shield him from the hot afternoon sun, the caregiver holds an umbrella over Dad's legs as the rabbi begins the short ceremony. He summarizes Mom's life with a lovely lyrical quality. First my son speaks. Then my niece speaks. I say a few words and relay the message from my Dad about how happy her trip was back to Germany with him many years prior. Lastly my brother speaks about our mother and thoughtfully recalls her resilience in making a new life for herself in America after she was forced to leave behind her loving family and the home in Germany that she adored.

As we rise for the Kaddish and the lowering of the casket into the grave, my father takes off his wedding ring and hands it to me to ask for it to be placed in the casket. The funeral attendants find a way to place the ring in the casket.

We return to our house and are comforted by a smattering of friends and family and especially by our grandchildren who add some levity to the sobriety of the day. It's Friday night and we light the candles and say the blessings over the bread and wine. We are all together to comfort one another. Even Dad puts his feet up, drinks a bit of wine and eats the dinner. Though we are sad at Mom's passing, we are relieved that she is out of her misery. My brother adds a bit of his cynical humor to the occasion. He thinks Dad held out. "It's always been a contest," he says.

Dad wants to know where he will be buried. "Right next to Mom," I assure him.

Tying Things Up

A few days after the funeral, we go to Mom's unit to close things up. I bring a big tray of cookies to show my appreciation to the staff for all they have done for Mom. The staff presents me with several of her paintings and tells me she had been a runner-up for the Alzheimer's Association "Memories in the Making" event.

We sort out the clothes and furniture and have a charity come and pick up some of it. Our mover Ed takes the remaining items back to our house to store in our now bulging basement.

I notify all the legal and financial entities of Mom's death. This requires a list of phone calls and then consequently mailing out death certificates.

Note to self: Believe that Mom's dementia unit where she spent her final year was more than likely the best part of Mom and Dad's move to Denver. Mom had been living like a vegetable in Chicago but in a short amount of time and with the encouragement of the staff at Elm Place, she was able to adapt and embrace her new surroundings until she was no longer with us.

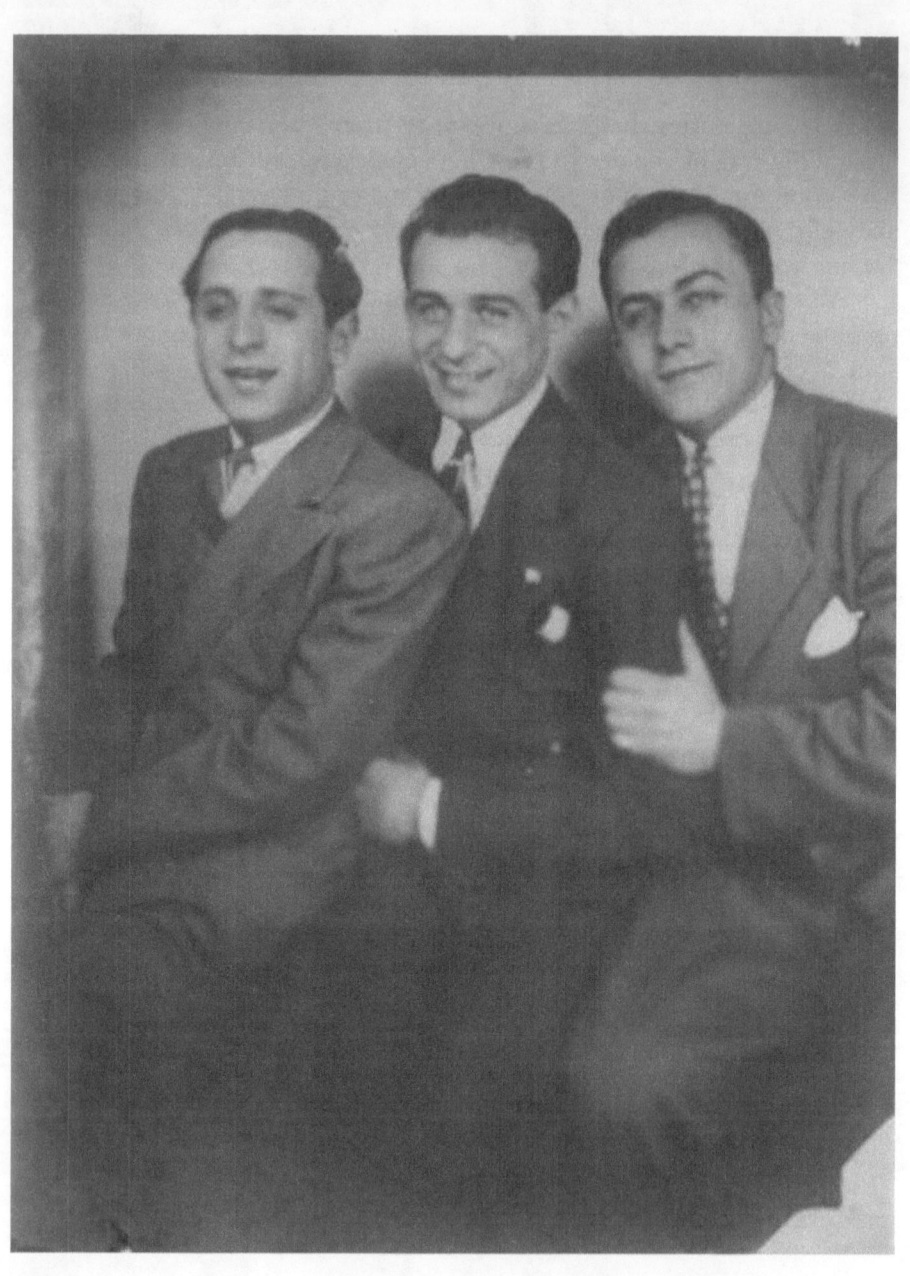

Chapter Nineteen

Dad's Last Days

Wheeling Dad to the gardens near Oak Tree, buying him lemonade from a little girl on the corner of one of the cross streets, admiring the signs of spring with him, we are taking each day as it comes.

March to June 2012

Trying to Make the Best of Things

Dad is becoming more and more needy. Each day he is dressed by a caregiver and offered some breakfast of which he eats very little. When I arrive he is seated in his recliner and usually dozing with the tubes from the oxygen tank inserted into his nostrils.

He'll wake up and say hi and then doze off soon after. I, usually in my running clothes, will then go through his closet, take his dirty shirts that must go to the cleaners and then count how many pants are hanging to make sure there are enough for the week.

We finally have a personalized daily living plan for Dad. That took at least two weeks to be determined. Once again I have met with the hospice team, this time to discuss Dad. The meeting takes place while we are awaiting Mom's funeral.

Most afternoons I meet my husband at Dad's apartment. On nice days we put Dad in the wheelchair with his portable oxygen unit and take him for walks to the nearby park. Dad has directed us to bring wine to his apartment, which we do each day, and then we stay until Dad's dinner arrives. Exhausted from the day's activities and Dad's current state, after he has finished his dinner, we go home and try to relax.

Every day I write out the sports schedule for Dad so he will know when the Cubs and Sox are playing and though Dad has no interest in the Rockies, I write out the schedule for them as well. Dad is also very fond of golf and he and my husband often watch the weekend matches. He loves bonding with my husband.

I've called the Jewish Family Service to see if I can find a Jewish companion for Dad. There's a lot of paperwork involved and a lot of time lapses in between the process.

The Jewish Family Service has finally found a companion for Dad and he visits Dad in addition to the hospice spiritual counselor's Mom. Dad's favorite companion is Marty, the hospice nurse who bathes and grooms him. She's getting married in August and Dad wants to be invited to the wedding. She brings him an invitation.

I've decided to hire someone twice a week in the afternoon to spell my husband and I from our tedious routine. After calling Sonia, the missing geriatric manager, several times, I give up. I contact Sally, the social worker from the other service I initially interviewed who, at the time, didn't seem to be the appropriate fit as a geriatric care manager. She assures me that she can perform any duties that I need and admits that she initially had underplayed her company's ability to perform the role of care manager. Luckily she turns out to be much more professional than our missing care manager. There is only a little bit of paperwork to do before Tonya arrives each Tuesday and Thursday afternoon. On nice days she takes Dad for a walk or downstairs for a drink. It's an activity and it works well.

They have begun working on our mountain bathrooms.

Dad is now the center of my life. He is not eating and is extremely weak. His diet is now reduced mainly to liquids. Each day I try to get through my exercise routine before stopping at Burger King to pick up a strawberry milk shake for Dad's lunch. I have stocked his refrigerator with different flavors of Ensure. Elena, one of Dad's most devoted caregivers in AL, has suggested all kinds of vitamins to put in Dad's liquids to make him stronger. I try them all. I buy colorful straws for Dad to use. I do anything I can think of to try to cheer him up and make him eat.

Again, this month as for the past several months, I have missed my book club and my lunch group. I always intend to go and then have to cancel. I've talked to none of my friends since I have taken over as caregiver to my parents. The only people I speak to regularly are my father's cousins from California, my brother and periodically my parents' friends. My husband and my children are really my mainstay. It's a bit lonely out there, but really there's no time for anything more.

April 2012

I've been trying to take care of myself. I've been very forgetful. I even forgot to RSVP to a bar mitzvah invitation. That's totally unlike me. Today a friend invited me in for a visit when I was returning something to her. It actually felt good to just relax for a while.

Oak Tree is having a Sedar for Passover and Dad says he wants to go. In honor of the Sedar, I get my nails done, one of the few acts I can think of to cheer myself up. Pretty bad when the only event you're attending is a senior residential Sedar.

We all get dressed up for the occasion. Dad makes it through the dinner but only manages to eat a sip of soup. The company is delightful and quite diverse. One elderly woman in IL is there with her kooky niece who is caring for her; another independent lady from IL is there by herself, and another woman my age is there with her mother. We're a very amicable group. The rabbi from Jewish Family Service conducts the service and even asks me to read an excerpt. The food is great. Though Dad was reluctant at the last moment to follow through on attending and though we don't make it to dessert, I actually think he has a good time.

Dad's friend Hank from Chicago has come out to visit with Dad and with his children who live in Denver. His wife had died in December right before Mom passed away. Every day of his three-day visit he comes with his children to briefly see Dad. Dad is too weak to dine with us but is elevated by his best friend's company. Every day that Hank comes, he addresses Dad like they were back playing bridge together. "Hey Leonard," he'll say. "We're having trouble finding someone to take over your place at bridge." Or he'll talk about the temple's troubles that have been going on for years. "I don't know if they've got enough new blood to take over," he'll say. He regales Dad with his workout routine. Not bad for a ninety-two year old. Hank is special. His gift is that he always has a twinkle in his eye and he addresses each moment as if it were the only one. His daughter and son-in-law are amenable to the process and join in easily.

My brother flies in to Denver on his way down to Albuquerque to check on the house they are building which is now close to completion. I let him take over for a while. He takes Dad for a walk to the park nearby where my husband and I walk him frequently. The spring flowers are beginning to bloom and Dad takes great pride in pointing them out. We're hoping he'll be able to see the gardens in full bloom this summer.

One Sunday I run the annual five-kilometer Cherry Creek Sneak and then my husband and I walk down to visit Dad. We are so lucky to have such great weather in Denver. It makes the predictability of each day much easier to handle.

One of Dad's nieces whom he has not spoken to in a very long time begins to contact us frequently. She writes long e-mails to me and sends several packages to Dad. This occupies all of us. One of the packages is filled with individually wrapped cookies in several flavors that she bakes for a living. She also sends some of her father's baseball books. Periodically Dad looks up to see me going through the wrappings. It's an activity. We strew the books on the coffee table knowing that they will not get read.

May 2012

Mostly our days are filled with a sameness, a concern that Dad is comfortable, that he's being tended to and that he is not in pain. More than that I'm not sure what to do. With the exception of one day, when he falls out of bed, he is in a holding pattern.

Every day I have confrontations with the staff. Some of this could be because I'm on edge and just not being very tolerant. Dad is not a very demanding person. We have given him a pendant and tried to teach him how to use it if he needs something, but he rarely uses it. We rely on hospice to check in on him, but unless there is some sort of emergency, they come only once or so a week. My rock is Elena. She's young and new and caring and she loves my dad. The other caregivers all have their problems. Noah takes his job very seriously but you have to tell him everything to do. Cassidy skips out a lot. Again, you have to tell her what Dad's needs are.

Periodically the children and the grandkids visit Dad. They always bring a smile to Dad. "She's a doll," he says of our daughter-in-law.

Regularly I see members of the hospice team as they make their rounds and as I am coming and going to see Dad. They give me a current report, which goes all over the place. One day one nurse thinks Dad is coming down with pneumonia. The next day another nurse checks him and says he's fine. Rosemary, the social worker, is concerned about me. She's always asking me to meet with her and, though I say I will, I never call. I'm just not one to break down with anyone unless they really probe.

Finally Rosemary and I make an appointment for the Friday after Father's Day to talk about how to tell Dad that I give him permission to die. I have been unable to do this mostly because I just can't. I love my Dad and though I have done little to proactively bring him back to a vigorous state, I just really can't acknowledge that I'm ready for him to give in.

Dad is getting weaker and weaker and eating less and less. For the first time he stays in bed all day. The next day he feels better and is up again.

June 2012

It's June and my cousin Sadie wants to come to Denver from LA and say good-by to Dad. She asks me what I think and I tell her to do what feels comfortable. Lately, in addition to the caregivers that visit Dad twice a week, I have hired caregivers for the night shift too just to be sure that Dad's needs are met. If he is going to die soon, I don't want him to be alone.

Sadie comes on Friday of Father's Day weekend. My Dad gives her a big smile when she walks into his room. He is in bed today and on Saturday as well.

The End

On Father's Day, my husband, my cousin Sadie and I arrive and Dad is again sitting in his chair. We give Dad a card that I've bought and a silly *National Geographic* CD that doesn't work. Dad reads the schmaltzy card and loves it. Why can't I express my feelings like the card does?

In the late afternoon my cousin and I come by once more and Dad is in bed again, but he opens his eyes when we arrive. He seems happy to see us. I tell him that my brother and his family are on their way to Denver to move permanently into their almost completed new home in Albuquerque and that they will be here on Tuesday. Then we both take turns saying good-by. I have a cold so I don't want to kiss Dad. I take his hand instead. He gives me an extra squeeze. "See you tomorrow," I say. The nurse calls at 8:30 to give me a report on Dad, which seems kind of strange. At 12:30 the next morning I get the final call. Dad is finally at peace.

I call my brother immediately. He is caravanning with his family in two cars packed with all the belongings they have not put on the moving truck to Albuquerque. Somehow or another the rest of the night passes and the next morning on Monday, the arrangements for another funeral begin again.

Another Funeral

Having had some recent experience in planning a funeral, preparations seem to flow a little bit easier this time. I notify the funeral home, try to get the same rabbi again who first says yes and then says no because he's moving to Connecticut the next week. Then, because our rabbi has expressed an interest in coming to Denver from the mountains to conduct Dad's funeral, I call her and she says she will be pleased to do the ceremony. My husband

and I make the funeral arrangements since my brother is in transit. I call the caterer, the florist, a server and things move rapidly from there. This time only our younger son from LA needs to fly in. We all have a conference call with the rabbi on Tuesday. The funeral is scheduled for Thursday afternoon. My brother and his family arrive the day before and again stay with us. Our younger son stays with his brother.

The ceremony is in many ways a repeat of Mom's, but in some ways a bit different. First of all, the rabbi is a lot more observant. Mom would have never approved, but since Dad always said he was an atheist and since none of it mattered to Dad as long as it was a Jewish ceremony, I think he would have thought it was fine. This time the younger grandchildren speak. The rabbi summarizes Dad's life and my brother and my husband and I each speak briefly.

This time my husband notifies his friends and associates and along with a few local friends and relatives in attendance, the graveside ceremony is just a bit larger than Mom's but still small and intimate.

We all gather at our house afterwards for dinner. The grandkids come again and some of our children's friends and family come as well. It is good to have the support.

The next day my husband and I go up to the mountains for the first time since March when Mom died, and my brother and his family stay at our home in Denver to get some R and R and to pack up some of Dad's belongings before they continue journeying on to Albuquerque.

On the Monday after the weekend, for the final time we call Ed, the mover, and have him deliver the rest of Dad's belongings downstairs to our basement in Denver. At this point our basement looks like a candidate for a rummage store.

Dad had died only three months after Mom and only a year and a month after they had moved to Denver. I took umbrage in the fact that my father told me when Mom died that he was happy they had made the move and that he had no regrets. I think my Dad had held out dying as long as he had because Mom was his responsibility and when he knew he could pass that duty on to me, he could rest peacefully. He told one of the nurses who took care of him that he "had had a good life." After all of the anxiety he felt at the time of Mom's death, he had finally put his concerns to rest.

Now we could plan to give both Mom and Dad a worthy tribute in Chicago. That would be the most memorable way of all to say good-by. The memorial would take place in August among all their legions of friends, many who had kept in contact with them even after they had moved to Denver.

Note to self: It's interesting to have watched the process of dying occur in both Mom and Dad. One day they were up and the next day back in bed. I'm beginning to become aware that the natural evolution in the process of dying is for this to occur. It makes me more aware of what to expect when my own time comes.

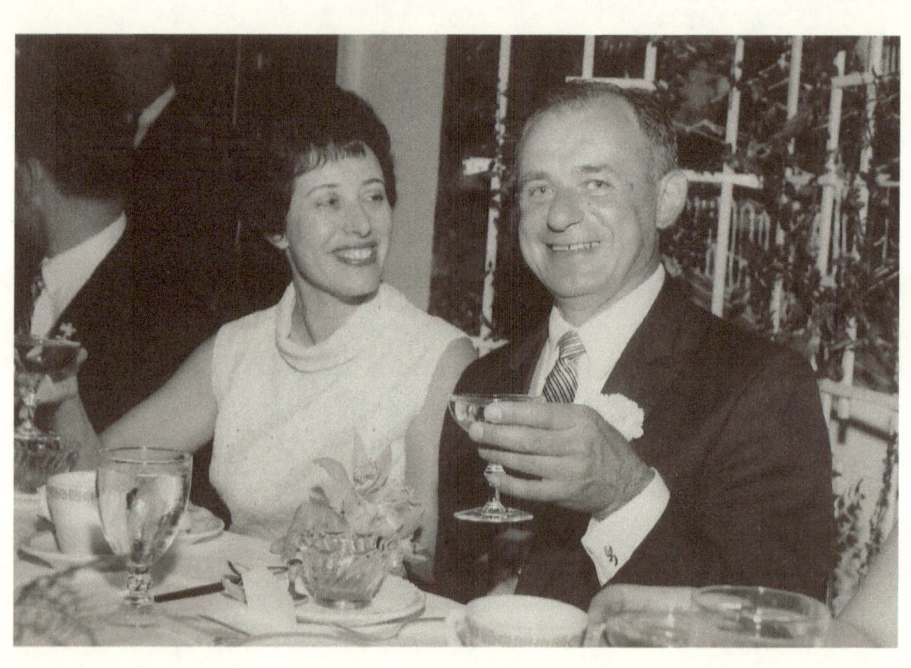

Chapter Twenty

The Memorial

How could I not love returning to Mom and Dad's community and reveling in their memories with so many people I have known all my life? This is great closure.

Taking Care of Business

There is so much follow-up to do: move Dad's belongings out of Oak Tree and back to our house, order a headstone for Mom and Dad's graves, write thank you notes to all of the people who have donated in Dad's memory or who have sent cards, take care of bills, cancel subscriptions, end agreements with Oak Tree, notify the insurance companies, Social Security and Medicare, and the financial advisor who manages Mom and Dad's affairs. My father at 95 was meticulous with his personal affairs but the finalizing of all the details still needs to be tended to. It takes several readings of Dad's will to get everything straight and then more time to carry through on his wishes.

Again, each day has been limited to just the necessities, i.e. working out, babysitting with the grandkids, and taking care of business. Our summer concert season has started in the mountains and we will be going up every weekend for the series. I am not really ready to socialize much with people. I'm still very tentative, sort of not in this world.

Getting Ready for the Memorial

We schedule Mom and Dad's memorial in Chicago for immediately after the concert season. I make up invitations and send them out to at least fifty people. I speak with the rabbi long distance about Mom and Dad. She schedules yet another conference call for my brother and me. I get in touch with the temple administrator who helps me plan the reception that will follow the memorial. Friends of ours have graciously invited us to stay with them in downtown Chicago for the weekend. Just my brother and my husband and I will be attending. We have told the children that it's not necessary for them to come. After all they have recently been to two funerals. My sister-in-law stays in their new home in Albuquerque rather than make a trip that would be very difficult for her considering her state of health.

In addition to the rabbi's eulogy, I have asked two of my mom and dad's best friends to recall some of their favorite memories. They have graciously consented to speak.

I put together a program to distribute at the service. The program has a picture of Mom and Dad on the front cover and the dates of their births and deaths. Inside is a copy of the poem, "Life is a Journey," that is frequently recited at the Jewish funeral service and is a favorite of my husband's and mine. For those who will attend the funeral, I have written a short synopsis of Mom and Dad's "Last Year" of their journeys and have included the Hebrew and English translation of the Kaddish, the final words that are repeated at the time of death.

Both my brother and I put together our own consolidated photo albums of Mom and Dad's lives, i.e. Mom's home in Germany, Dad's family in sepia and then all of the photos of their courtship, their honeymoon, their friends, their trips and even some of us although we humorously think we have the least amount of pictures. My niece had put together a book of pictures of Mom and Dad with their friends and all of the trips they took for them to have in Denver, and I pack that up as well.

I am nervous about having the memorial but I really feel that I want to do it for my parents' friends. They have been so wonderful to Mom and Dad even after they moved to Denver. They need some closure too. But how many people will be there? I tell the caterer at the most fifty, but more likely thirty.

Memorial Day

The day arrives, a lovely Chicago summer day, and we arrive early to set things up. Again there are flowers (blue and white, my mother's favorite colors); again there is a helper to make sure everything gets done; again there is food, this time lox and bagels and lots of pastries which my mom would have loved although maybe not so much because I ordered them and she didn't bake them!

The service takes place in the synagogue that my parents helped to build with their money, their energy and their passion. It is where I was confirmed, where I was married and where our children were named.

At the entrance to the synagogue, my brother, my husband and I greet the many people whose lives have touched both my parents and us as well, way more than fifty of them. So many friends, some still couples, some widows, some widowers, some ailing, some still in good shape, but all resilient, positive and delightful. There are contemporaries of Mom and Dad's in their late eighties and nineties, several children of their friends now in their fifties and sixties, a few relatives of my mother's, people Mom and Dad have known through the temple, some of Dad's acquaintances he has known through business and through his activities in the community, their neighbor for over thirty years, relatives of my husband's and friends of both my brother and mine. I have asked them all to sign a guest book. Later I count them. There are eighty people. What a tribute to my parents!

Before the service the rabbi takes my husband and I to an alcove where memorial plaques are displayed and where we will soon have one for Mom and Dad. She shows us a large Bible beautifully illustrated in gold fill that my father had given to the temple. She is so pleased with his gift and wants us to know about Dad's donation.

The service begins. My brother welcomes everyone and thanks everyone for coming.

Then Ruth comes up to the pulpit. She is still walking tentatively after recently breaking her ankle. She talks about all the wonderful times she has had with Mom and Dad, about what a gracious hostess Mom was and about her beautiful manners.

Then Hank gets up and talks about being friends with Mom and Dad, all the places they traveled together and all the holidays and special occasions they shared. He even reveals a fact that I never knew about my mom, that as a child she was driven to school in a limousine. He also talks about a visit to South Carolina, the home of his late wife's non-Jewish family and the culture clash that occurred when Mom and Dad met them.

The rabbi then recounts the key moments of Mom and Dad's lives, particularly their vital contribution to the temple.

At the end it's my turn to speak and invite everyone into the community hall to have some brunch and to have them share some of their own stories about Mom and Dad. I am extremely moved as I face the sea of familiar faces.

On each of the tables I have placed a picture of Mom and Dad at different times in their lives. Along with the albums, they provide great fodder for recalling stories of Mom and Dad.

To think that at the end of their very long lives, my mother and father could still leave such a lasting legacy was profound to me. All those years when I just wanted to rebel and get away and become independent may have been important but at the end my respect and admiration for them both continues to grow. How they dealt with adversity, particularly that which one can face at the end of life, is truly something to honor.

Note to self: My parents' friends' memories have enriched my understanding of my parents more than I ever could have imagined. Do you think people younger than I will think that way of me????

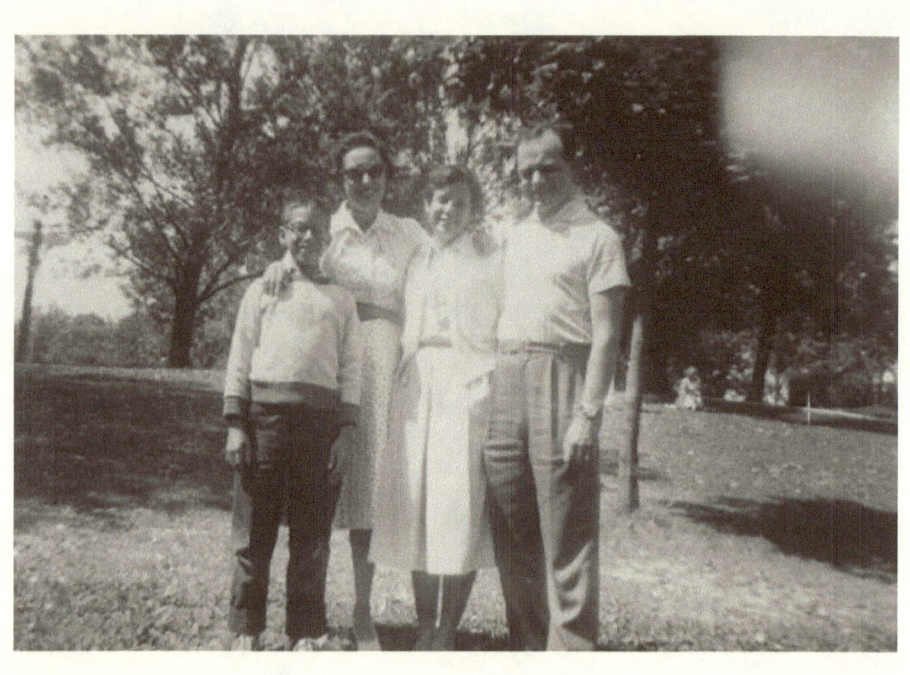

Chapter Twenty-One

Mourning

OK, so Mom and Dad had their issues. Don't we all? They're looking better and better all the time. Can you believe it's working out this way?

It took a year before the finality of being an "orphan" settled in.

The immediate aftermath really did not allow much time for mourning. We, of course had to clean out Mom's and Dad's residences and dispose of as much as we could of their personal belongings. A year and a half later a great amount of their belongings still are housed in our basement. I am vowing to take care of this as soon as I finish this book.

I really didn't begin to have some down time until after the memorial that we held for Mom and Dad's friends in August in Chicago.

Most of the summer after Dad passed away was spent attending concerts in the mountains and caring for our grandchildren in the city. It was good to stay busy and just take one day at a time.

A couple of months after the memorial, I returned to my monthly girls' lunch and to my book club. Beyond that I found my greatest comfort from my family. I still felt when I was with other people that I was not quite in the real world.

All my extra energies went into helping with the national election that was coming up in November. I threw myself into making phone calls, manning their office and doing whatever they asked me to do.

For Thanksgiving, my husband and I headed down to Albuquerque to be with my brother and his family in their new green home. Being together without having to worry about Mom and Dad was very strange, like there was a big empty hole. We didn't have to have Mom's giblet stuffing or her awful sweet potatoes. We could have guacamole for an appetizer and our own choice of vegetables and salad. (Mom never cooked a fresh vegetable and she only liked iceberg lettuce.) I met that freedom with mixed emotions.

In February my brother and his wife came up to Denver to be with us for the dedication of Mom and Dad's headstone. My cousin officiated at the very small ceremony that was followed by a small family dinner.

Made of Colorado marble, the dual headstone reads:

Liese Henle Rothman	Leonard Rothman
December 25, 1920-March 12, 2012	December 27, 1915-June 18, 2012

"Life is a Journey"

In between the name of my parents is carved Mom and Dad's temple logo of a burning bush.

On the anniversary of both Mom and Dad's deaths, my husband and I attend Friday night services and light a candle for each of them.

Then it is finally time to move on and to fill the gap that had been so occupied for the past year with the constant care of Mom and Dad since they were with us in Denver.

No day goes by when I am not reminded of something that connects me to each of my parents. I pass the gardens where my husband and I used to walk Dad and it makes me wish Dad could have seen it when it was in full bloom. I pass the pastry shop where I purchased key lime tartlets for them both and chuckle at how much they both relished that dessert. I go to Target and see a motorized cart and remember when Dad drove it down the toy aisle to select a birthday gift for his great-grandson.

Though at the beginning of the mourning period, I felt the sting of their absence more intensely, as time passes, the memories come and go in a more soft and impressionistic manner.

As time passes too, I become more and more aware of the legacy Mom and Dad left my brother and I. There's a great deal of comfort in having this legacy in common with him and in being able to talk about it. More than anything, I think my father instilled in both of us a responsibility to take care of our family. I think my mother, although our relationship was always rocky, turned out to be a pretty sunny lady despite all the adversity she was forced to face. And wow! Did she give us an unusual European perspective to blend into our totally suburban upbringing! I think I also realize my parents' liabilities as well and hope to learn from those too. My mother was dogmatic and harsh in her beliefs; my father was often too principled and way too inclined to wear his heart on his sleeve.

When my husband and I went to Israel recently, it seemed timely to be going the year after my Mom and Dad passed away and to visit this country for the first time in our lives. There were so many reminders there of memories and messages my parents whether intentionally or subliminally passed on to me. I couldn't help think of my father's parents, both Russian immigrants, who were early Zionists and supported the founding of Israel unlike my mother who was against it. At the Israel Museum we saw silver artifacts just like those my mom brought to America from Germany and sculptures by modern artists like Henry Moore and Giacometti whom my mom revered. And, of course, we visited Yad Vashem, the Holocaust Museum that chronicled a period of time that was germane to my mother's life and that totally ruled how she and our family existed.

When I got back to Denver, I went through some of Mom's old papers just to see how much of her secretive life before she came to America I could unveil. It's going to take some real intention if this is ever to occur.

The other surprise when I got home was a discovery of all her travel diaries. In the process of moving, they had been buried in a container in one of the closets downstairs in the basement. If I had been younger, I would have never wanted to look at them, but now they were very meaningful. She had two on Israel. Mostly they were about shopping!!!

Note to self: Though their time in Denver was short before they passed away, it was a good year for everyone. We all made the most of the little time that was left and I think we all feel good about that. As my father said, there are no regrets.

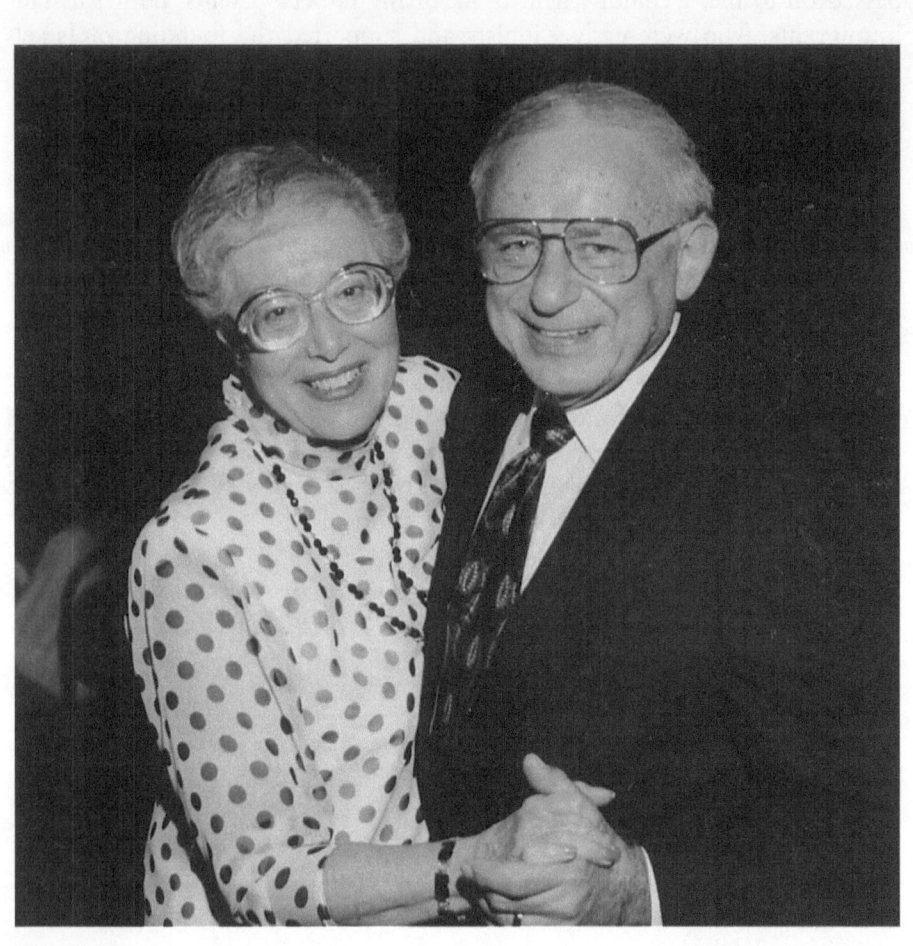

Chapter Twenty-Two

Reflections

So I did the best I could. It may not have been perfect, but I tried. On balance, I think I did all right.

My decision to move my parents here at the ages of 90 and 95 was a personal one and not particularly conventional. I do my best to convince myself that I made all the right decisions, but I can't help looking back and reflecting on those choices mostly because I'm a Libra and I always look at both sides of the story, but also because these same questions will come up as my husband and I begin to age.

None of us is perfect and we all do what we think is right and then we need to learn to live with it. I am content that in the case of the decisions that I made for my parents, I did my very best to make them as comfortable as possible in their very old age.

On a selfish note, I am grateful that my parents were with me for their last year. I am so sad that they didn't stay longer.

I am impressed by my parents' tenacity and courage.

I am overwhelmed by the support given to me by my husband, my children, my brother and sister-in-law, and the myriads of people who cared about Mom and Dad during this period of time.

Denver vs. Chicago

I take great solace in the fact that my father once said to me near the end of his life that he had no regrets about moving to Denver and that together we had made the right decision.

I wish I had known more about how people age and how difficult it is for most to adjust to anything new. That might have forced me to try harder to keep them in their familiar environment. On the other hand, even if they had initially remained in their original homes, at some point a large portion of elderly people are forced to change locations anyway.

The upside of the choices I made is that my parents continued to have adventures and that they probably had a much better quality of life in their last year than they would have had if they had stayed in Chicago.

Housing Choices

I wish that Mom and Dad could have lived forever in their comfortable suburban home. That would definitely have been my first choice. The extenuating circumstances made this reality impossible. The maintenance of the house became an issue. Where they lived made them a target for intruders. Despite the additional help of a housekeeper/caregiver, it was difficult for them to get through the day with any joy. Perhaps I could have found ways to compensate for these problems, but I feel I did my best and keeping them in their home just didn't work.

The selection of the first continuing care facility was based on Mom and Dad's preferences rather than mine and I feel this was appropriate. I do dwell occasionally on my decision to place them in separate bedrooms. My reasoning was based on the fact that Mom's needs were so different than Dad's and yet I wanted to keep them together.

I felt that Mom's aggressiveness and disorientation was impossible for both Dad and the caregivers to handle. I sometimes think her behavior was exacerbated by separating them and that perhaps I should have placed them together and seen if that would have worked out better. I really doubt that. I've done a lot of reading about eldercare and though it is true that elder people with dementia often act out because of frustration, some of their behavior is based on their psychological roots and their personality traits. Mom was not by nature a soft and gentle person and her sad family history had forced her to be tough and combative.

I am particularly satisfied with my decision to place Dad in independent housing and Mom in a dementia unit when they moved to Denver and to have kept them in the same complex near my residence. Considering that I had to address the concerns of Mom, Dad and me, I did the best I could and it worked for a while.

All the changes that took place after Mom and Dad began to have more health problems were knee-jerk reactions to situations that needed resolution quickly. Looking back, I think that I might have done better if I had known more about all the options available. If I had had more knowledge, I might have considered a nursing home for both of them as their problems increased. As it turned out, the other options seemed to have served them relatively well.

As far as type of facility, I believe that my choices reflected my values. I like a corporate environment even though there are many drawbacks and flaws in their operations. I have friends who are much happier with locally owned facilities or even not for profit facilities. For me this was the right choice.

Caregiving

I am glad I was the caregiver in charge but I am also very glad that I was able to hire people to assist in the caregiving process.

I have the utmost regard for good caregivers, but I also realize that, like teachers do not all have the same abilities, neither do caregivers.

My strength as a caregiver was more in organizing and getting things done than it was in nurturing. I dutifully performed my obligations but not always with heart. In retrospect I wish I could have been more open and emotional, but I did the best I could. Certainly I have no regrets about being attentive. In fact, as the hospice team often suggested, I needed to separate myself from my parents more frequently and to give myself some space. I think in the long run I did take time out for myself and I knew when things were getting to me and I did leave the scene for a while when I seemed to be "losing it."

We Are All Different

Dealing with two parents at the same time forced me to realize how different the aging process is for each person and how different personalities cope.

Physically Dad was in much better shape than Mom who could not talk and who had lost many more of her mental faculties than Dad, but Mom took things in stride where Dad was always discontent. Mom was much more independent in her needs and Dad was much more reliant on us to occupy him and to lift him out of his doldrums. I think it was difficult on both of them that the other was not around, but that is sometimes the cruelty of old age.

I tried to deal with each of them as individuals. For Mom just being there seemed to suffice. For Dad I felt I always had to try to cheer him up and make him less needy. At the age of 96, the reality was that change was not likely to happen.

It is interesting to me now that my parents have passed to theorize about personality traits I might have missed, but alas it's too late to take them into consideration. Maybe Mom was more cognizant than I realize. Maybe Dad would have never been happy no matter where I placed him. So be it.

Money Matters

In this book I wished only to explain how I took care of my parents in a personal way and to say that, regardless of one's financial strata, almost all of us worry about money and so many other issues as well.

I feel very fortunate that my parents provided enough means to care for them with assistance. Had this fact not been the case, I am very aware of how much more difficult and time-consuming my duties would have been.

I am pleased with my money management. At times it was very frustrating to handle all of the bills and insurance issues and to make decisions on where and where not to spend money, but in the long run I have few regrets.

Medical Decisions

I chose to have a geriatrician make my parents' medical decisions rather than selecting a primary care doctor and hiring specialists for my parents' various medical problems. I believe a geriatrician has more experience in realizing what is normal about how the elderly age and what are their needs. I think there are probably geriatricians out there who would have been more aggressive about medicating their patients than the doctor I chose, but I was pleased with his approach.

I do think that I had to be assertive sometimes when Dr. Higby was not so as in the case of medicating Dad for depression and of pursuing hospice for Mom, but to me that was a part of my job as caregiver. The doctor wasn't there everyday to carefully monitor my parents' needs. If I hadn't been in the same city with them, that would have been a problem.

I do think that I learned to listen and to go with my own gut when I had to make decisions. I was happy to hear others' thoughts, but in the long run Mom and Dad were my responsibility and I made the calls.

There Comes a Time

The whole time that I was taking care of my parents I was concerned more with making each day worthwhile rather than sustaining life just for the sake of living. I was willing to lessen Mom's medications so she would be alert even though I knew that this would decrease her longevity. With Dad, I did not force-feed him when he lost his interest in eating nor did I ask the doctor to feed him intravenously. I often think about the Native American tradition where an elder when he is ready to die goes out to the fields and chants until his time comes. I feel my parents knew how much I enjoyed them and I tried constantly to give them things to look forward to, but I felt in the long run it was their choice to determine whether they would like to go on living. Sometimes I feel I didn't give them enough motivation for continuing on, but I also console myself by acknowledging that they knew they were being taken care of and could relax enough to decide.

Life is a Journey

Though for over one year I was on caregiving duty every day, I do not resent the time I spent taking care of Mom and Dad. They took care of me when I was growing up and when it was my turn to take care of them, I was very happy to do so. I feel that I did the best that I could and most of the time I think I did a pretty good job. I guess you could say that they are at peace and I am at peace too.

Note to self: Never again do you have to feel that your roots are not worthy of recognition. This entire experience should remind you of how life can be creative and memorable. You have at the most fifteen years left before you will be in the same situation as your mom and dad were (if you're lucky) so make the most of it and prepare as much as you can. You have good role models to follow.

Acknowledgments

I'd like to thank all the people who helped me take care of Mom and Dad. I could never have done this on my own.

I'd like to thank all of Mom and Dad's wonderful friends who continued to stay in touch even after Mom and Dad had moved to Denver.

I'd like to thank my friend, Jan Lewis, a fellow writer, for using her fine skills to guide me in my efforts to write this book.

I'd like to thank my friend, Barbara Bronner, who lent her expertise as a geriatric social worker to assure my accuracy on that subject.

I'd like to thank my son Adam for helping me "package" the book.

I'd like to thank my brother Mick who intimately knows this subject matter and whose writing and editing commentary were extremely helpful.

Finally, I'd like to thank my husband who was my constant companion during this entire time period and who, though he may not have liked revisiting this experience so soon after it happened, took the time to read and review the book.

Appendix I

Mimi's Ten Commandments Of Eldercare

I. *Analyze your personal circumstances*

   a. Try to define the physical, mental and emotional state of the particular individual you are caring for.
   b. Consider the elderly person's ability to make rational decisions.
   c. Take into account that everyone's situation is different and that there is no norm.
   d. Consider all the personalities involved if you can, both on the caregiver side and on the side of the aging person.
   e. Assess how decisions are made in your family, and, if at all possible, either put someone in charge, assume the responsibilities yourself, or farm out the responsibilities to someone else.

II. *Prioritize*

   Based on your assessments, what is most important for the aging person and the caregiver? Safety? Quality of Life? Logistics of the caregiver? Least hassle for the caregiver? Medical issues? Financial issues?

III. *Stay Fluid*

   Have an idea of where you are going, but also be prepared to switch gears if a crisis occurs or there are signals that warrant considering a change.

IV. *Educate Yourself*

It's good to have some sort of general overview of the entire eldercare scene and then to zero in on the issue at hand when the time comes to address that particular subject.

V. *Communicate with everyone.*

No matter who you're dealing with, your loved ones, your children, your siblings, your doctors, your caregivers, you need to take the time to hear where they're coming from and to respond in a positive, upbeat manner. After all, you're in this together so you might as well try to get along.

VI. *Learn every bureaucracy and deal with each one of them individually.*

The ER has one set up, assisted living has another structure, caregivers have another model. Every structure is organized differently and you have to figure out how to navigate through each one of them. Sometimes it's by going to the boss; sometimes you have to go above the boss to another boss. It's complicated.

VII. *Stand Your Ground*

Tell people if something needs to get done, i.e. the laundry, the pills, whatever, but try to sugar coat it without pointing any fingers.

VIII. *Organize*

Make sure that all contracts are at your fingertips when you need to figure out how long they are in place before changes can be made. Make sure you have all the important data for your loved one available in case someone requests that information. Make sure too that you leave enough time to take care of bills, see your charges regularly and allow enough time to relax in between.

IX. *Do Your Homework*

That means leave as little to chance as possible. If your loved one suffers from depression, read up on how to cope with it so that you can ask intelligent questions of your doctor. If you're looking at housing, make sure you know what criteria you should consider and be sure to prepare a careful list of alternatives. The more you know about the situation, the more likely you are to act in a prudent way.

X.   *Take Care of Yourself*

Be sure to eat and sleep well, to exercise, and to take a little bit of time out to do something you want to do. And don't forget to keep your sense of humor. I used to amuse myself with playing only classical music on the radio to soothe my shattered nerves and I had fun making silly observations about the staff and the residents to myself. For example, I'd say to myself, "look at all those fancy canes" or "I wonder how many tons of Polident the residents use each year."

Appendix II

An Eldercare Primer

Based on my experiences and my subsequent research, here is my own attempt to simplify the very complicated world of eldercare.

An Overview

The best general terms with which to start a discussion are **eldercare** and **longterm care**.

Eldercare:
A wide range of services provided at home, in the community and in residential care facilities for people who are entering their later years.

Longterm Care:
This term is more concerned with the services needed in order for an elderly person to perform normal activities of daily living, which may be affected by diminishing abilities in cognitive skills or because of loss of muscular strength or control.

Where to Start

The **Administration on Aging**, which is part of the Department of Health and Human Services, is available to orient an individual on the most common aging and eldercare topics.

The **Area Administrations on Aging** are regional and state offices that disperse information on particular eldercare private and public services for specific communities.

Websites:

Go to **eldercarelocator.gov** for general information on services available nationally and locally.

Go to **longtermcare.gov** if you want to know how to qualify for governmental benefits.

Eldercare Topics

Below are some basic topics that come up regularly when discussing eldercare. They are a beginning point of reference and should lead the reader to all kinds of other options or links both public and private.

Housing: In-Home or Senior Living

In-Home

An elderly person makes a choice to remain in his home and to contract outside services for any extra needs. These outside services might be either based on professional *medical care* such as home health or based on *home support* such as caregiving, transportation, meals, home maintenance and recreational services.

Senior Living

In this situation, the elderly person moves to some sort of facility where his or her needs can be met in one place. Depending on the needs, seniors can choose from various types of facilities. They can be privately or publicly owned and include these options:

— Continuing Care Retirement Communities provide a variety of living options, usually independent living, assisted living, and skilled nursing care. As one ages, the resident can move from one unit to another without leaving the "Campus." Only the skilled care unit is government regulated.

— Independent Retirement Communities. These can be small or large complexes and financed in a variety of ways. In this environment, the elderly person lives in his own house, townhouse, condominium, apartment or other private unit which he either owns or rents. He conducts his own affairs but within the complex, he has access to all the services he needs currently and may need in the future. These facilities are not government regulated.

— Assisted Living Communities are a special combination of housing, personal services and health care designed to respond to the individual needs of those who require help with **Activities of Daily Living** such as bathing, dressing, toileting and mobility issues. Care is provided in a professionally managed group living environment and usually includes private occupancy units, three meals a day, 24-hour staff availability to meet the individual's scheduled and unscheduled needs and some medical care. These facilities have limited governmental regulations.

— Dementia Units are a form of assisted living facility that cares for people who have lost their ability to think cognitively. They are secured facilities but are considered a form of assisted living facility rather than a nursing facility. Many of these units are defined or specialized by their ability to take care of Alzheimer's patients.

— Skilled Care or Nursing Homes are less intensive facilities than hospital care and provide nursing and medical services. This type of facility is government regulated and can either be short term for recently hospitalized patients or more of a permanent set-up if the needs of the senior is more long term. Medicare pays for the short-term residence up to 100 days as long as the patient continues to "improve." Medicaid pays for longterm care if the patient qualifies. All nursing homes are government regulated and rated. See medicare.gov. Another payment option would be private pay.

— Respite Care is the provision of short-term, temporary relief to those who are caring for family members who might otherwise require permanent placement in a facility outside the home. This can be in the senior's home or at a senior facility.

— Hospice facilities. Residents who are not expected to live past six months can be placed in hospice facilities for which Medicare will pay. If they exceed the six months they must be transferred to another type of facility. An alternative to moving an elderly person to a hospice facility is to have hospice services administered in the current residence of the patient. Some hospice programs allow a patient to continue with hospice as long as the patient shows no signs of improvement even past the six-month period. Hospice does not pay for room and board.

— Adult Day Care services are provided during the day at a community-based center. Programs address the individual needs of functionally or cognitively impaired adults. These structured, comprehensive programs provide social and support services in a protective setting during any part of a day, but not 24-hour care. Many adult day service programs include health-related services. Many of these services offer financial aid in the community.

NOTES:
Both Medicare and Medicaid reimburse for care at the skilled nursing level if the resident qualifies and the facility has been certified by the nursing home standards. Only nursing homes can receive Medicaid assistance. Nursing homes that are accepted by Medicaid are listed under medicare.gov

Under Medicare.gov, the Centers for Medicare and Medicaid Services (CMS) evaluate nursing homes.

Assisted living facilities are not covered under Medicare or Medicaid but you can get a tax deduction because the resident must have assistance in his daily activities.

Regardless of what type of housing is selected, it is important to have in place an emergency plan. In some situations, this can be accomplished by purchasing pendants or emergency monitoring. Again, there is a wide range of possibilities.

Medical Care

Medical Care involves a network of licensed professionals who can perform all kinds of care for the elderly person.

Types of professionals involved include ***doctors, nurses, speech therapists, occupational therapists, physical therapists*** and many other certified assistants. All professionals must be licensed.

The network of services can be paid for privately or by Medicare and Medicaid. When the government pays for the services, the service must be a licensed **Provider**, i.e. a doctor, health care professional, hospital, home health agency or other health care facility.

Below are some medical services that the elderly person might use.

Hospitals

Medicare.gov lists those hospitals in your area that have the approval of the CMS (Center for Medicare and Medicaid Services). Hospitals included can be for profit or not for profit. It's a good idea to find out which hospital your doctor services and also to know which **emergency rooms** you might want to select should the need develop. You might want to ask the senior residence what their policy is on choosing a hospital.

Doctors

Doctors' qualifications and evaluations are sometimes quite confusing. Medicare.gov evaluates doctors that have the system's approval. If you go out of that network, you may want to see what kinds of payment and evaluation terms are available. Some of the more common alternative physician specialists you may be dealing with include:

— *Geriatricians*
Geriatricians are doctors who specialize in the needs of the elderly. The advantage of having a geriatrician care for the elderly patient is that they are particularly familiar with some of the types of problems the elderly person might experience such as common urinary tract infections, dementia, pneumonia, and depression. They generally have their own private practices but can service various senior residential facilities.

— *Emergency Room Doctors*
Seniors tend to wind up in emergency rooms for falls, infections, strokes, etc. An emergency room doctor often becomes a medical professional with whom the caregiver will need to interact. Sometimes you have a choice on where to send your loved one. Follow up care is done through Home Health (see Home Health topic) after the resident has been released from the ER or the hospital.

— *Specialists*
Specialists in diseases are frequently consulted while residents are aging such as cardiologists, neurologists, urologists, and oncologists. Consult medicare.gov to see if services by specialists are covered. In general this is not an area of coverage.

NOTES:

Medicare has a list of providers with whom they will work. Go to eldercarelocator.gov or longtermcare.gov or to medicare.gov.

Licensing for medical professionals is done in different ways, by the state and by the federal government. For example the U.S. Department of the Treasury licenses medical professionals nationally. In Colorado the Department of Public Health licenses medical facilities. One way to assess this complicated process is to see whether the service is a state or federal or county service.

Nurses

There are many kinds of nurses with different skills and education, which can be applied to many areas of eldercare. For example, nurses are used to administer home health aid, hospice care, work in assisted living and senior living residential facilities and to assist doctors. A nurse may earn advanced certification in areas such as psychiatric nursing. Basically, the kinds of nurses fall into several categories.

— *Registered Nurses (RN)* are graduate nurses who have completed a minimum of two years of education at an accredited school of nursing. RNs are licensed by the state in which they work. A Director of Nursing at a senior residence is usually an RN.

— *Licensed Practical Nurse (LPN)* are nurses who have completed one or two years in a school of nursing or vocational training school. LPNs are in charge of nursing in the absence of a Registered Nurse (RN). LPNs often give medications and perform treatments. They are licensed by the state in which they work.

— *Certified Nursing Assistants (CNA)* are trained and certified to help nurses by providing non-medical assistance to patients, such as help with eating, cleaning and dressing. The training can take place in a variety of places such as community colleges.

— *A Nurse Practitioners (NP)* are advanced practice registered nurses (APRN) who have completed advanced didactic and clinical education beyond that required of the generalist registered nurse (RN) role.

Technicians and Labs

May be independent providers and often bill Medicare, Medicaid and supplementary insurance companies separately. These services are normally performed in a hospital, a doctor's office or in the emergency room. They include the cost of lab tests and technicians.

Ambulance Services

You will probably deal with this service either because your senior called, or you or the caregiver called 911 or if your loved one is living in a senior facility, she may do the calling. A senior facility will use its own resources. If you call 911, you will use the designated service of that call. Both services are paid for by medicare.gov for the patient to be transported, but Medicare does not always pay for the return transport. Best to ask since you will probably be under extra pressure and won't have time to look up the rules.

Home Health Services

Home health includes the services of nurses, speech therapists, occupational therapists, and physical therapists and can either be performed in the patient's home or in a senior care facility. Under Medicare, home health services are provided to any senior who has been hospitalized or who has been sent to the emergency room. There are also many preventative home health services covered under Medicare and also available at many residential communities. Again, it's complicated and I suggest you ask a lot of questions or if you have several days, you can consult the website. A senior residential facility sometimes has its own home health unit to service their residences, which can be initially paid for by Medicare and then paid for privately. The patient is not required to use this specific service even if he is living in a senior facility that has such a unit.

— *Occupational Therapists (OT)* help the senior adapt to his environment after any kind of change in daily living.

— *Physical Therapists (PT)* are trained to retain or restore functioning in the musculature of the arms, legs, hands, feet, back and neck through movement, exercises or treatment.

— *Speech Therapists* are specialists in the evaluation and treatment of communication disorders and swallowing disorders.

NOTES:

Medicare.gov and longtermcare.gov both list approval ratings for home health agencies. Again there are many home health agencies and most of them are for profit, so they will need to be carefully screened.

Medical Equipment and Services

There are all kinds of medical equipment and service companies. These include oxygen companies, pharmaceutical service companies, companies that supply hospital beds, wheelchairs, etc. If you are living in a senior facility, it is more than likely that the facility will subcontract the service or purchase the equipment from one of their chosen purveyors. Sometimes the physician orders the company that will be used. If one is living independently, this may have to be done by the person overseeing the aging individual or the individual himself.

NOTES:

The government under Medicare pays for **Durable Medical Equipment**, i.e. medical equipment that is ordered by a doctor for use in the home. These items, such as walkers, wheelchairs, and hospital beds are required to be reusable. Durable medical equipment is paid for under Medicare, subject to a 20% coinsurance of the Medicare-approved amount.

Caregiving

A caregiver can be a family member, a volunteer or a paid employee who is taking care of an individual, in this case an elderly individual, who is in need of assistance in performing the tasks of daily life such as making and serving meals, bathing, dressing, dispensing medications, and assisting in any manner where the senior cannot perform his own tasks. Sometimes the caregiver's duties are companion or chauffeur. The duties are not structurally defined. At the moment the caregiving industry is limited in its governmental regulations.

Kinds of Caregivers

— *Family Caregiver* are members or friends who provide unpaid assistance to another adult who can no longer independently attend to his or her personal needs and/or perform his or her normal activities of daily living.

— *Independent Caregivers* either work privately during the day or live in and take care of a senior. They have a variety of experience and training. It's important to ask what are their credentials. It is also important to know that you will need to have them fill out tax forms.

— *Caregivers from Agencies*
The training and experience of both the head of the agency and the caregiver are variable. Again, it's good to ask what are the agency's credentials. Agencies will no doubt charge more than a private caregiver, but they will take care of taxes and hopefully make sure that you're getting a good quality caregiver.

— *Institutional Caregivers* are caregivers who take care of several residents on their shift and help feed, bathe and dress the residents and attend to their immediate needs. Even though senior residences often times have their own caregiving agencies, they will tend to be appropriate for more short term needs and will most likely not be as consistent as going through an agency if your loved one's needs are continual. In licensed facilities, caregivers are not allowed to give out medications unless they are certified nurse assistants. Again, ask what are the requirements of the caregivers the residence hires.

— *Geriatric Care Managers* are health care professional, typically a nurse or social worker, who arrange, monitor, or coordinate long-term care services (also referred to as a care coordinator or case manager). A care manager may also assess a patient's needs and develop a plan of care, subject to approval by the patient's physician. For more information, go to the National Association of Professional Geriatric Care Managers website at *http://www.caremanager.org*

NOTES:
There are many professional caregiver organizations that aim to establish criteria for caregiving but do not offer resources for finding caregivers. In our case, we found my parents' original caregiver through a referral. Initially I relied on the recommendations of the senior living facilities when my parents arrived in Denver. I tried the senior living residence's caregiving services but eventually hired caregivers from private companies recommended by a commercial referral agency.

Caregiver organizations perform a variety of functions from offering advice to providing information on financial assistance. Certification is variable. A good place to begin is the Family Caregiving Alliance National Center on caregiving *http://www.caregiver.org*

— *Housekeeping, Concierge and Other Services*

Sometimes caregivers are asked to perform housekeeping tasks as well as caregiving services. There's a lot of cross over between the two skills and sometimes if you get the right person, this can be the answer. The housekeeper/caregiver can be found in many ways such as through yellow pages, agencies, advertisements and referrals from friends.

Services that a caregiver might provide can also be contracted by the caregiver or the care manager or through a senior living facility. A few of those services that are needed by the elderly include beauty salons and barber shops, podiatrists, moving companies, grocery shopping services and transportation services. The area on aging website can often provide a beginning for pursuing these services. Sometimes local social service agencies can assist in this area.

NOTES:

Certification of caregivers, caregiver agencies and geriatric care managers vary from state to state and are somewhat arbitrary. It's important to ask what are the qualifications of those who are calling themselves caregivers or those operating an agency and also their years of experience in the business.

Many types of institutions offer certification for various aspects of caregiving. Hospitals will offer CPR courses; colleges will offer two to six month courses on caregiving, which will result in a certificate. One of the best ways for a caregiver to demonstrate her credentials is for her to take course work in becoming a certified nurse assistant that includes a state certification exam.

Eldercare.gov lists places where caregivers can become certified.

Caregiving also qualifies as a tax deduction by the federal government and in some states.

Financial Concerns Including Insurance and Medicare

Medicare and **Medicaid** are the two most frequently used sources for paying for the costly expenses of eldercare. (Medicare only absorbs the cost for those people over the age of sixty-five).

Medicare A (medicare.gov) pays a portion of hospital and doctor expenses if an elderly person is hospitalized. The expense is shared by the federal government and the state or region and may not cover all expenses. The statement often does not come for a long time. The statement will say **CMS,** Center for Medicare and Medicaid Services. The state or region will have a different name depending on where the elderly person lives.

Medicare B (medicare.gov) The government will partially pay for doctors' visits and some medical expenses in tandem with an insurance company that is contracted by the individual patient. Sometimes there may be a small additional co-payment. Big insurance companies like Aetna, Blue Cross Blue Shield and United Health Care are some of the companies available to policyholders depending on where one lives.

Medicare D (medicare.gov) pays for drugs oftentimes with co-payments that are supplemented by Medicare B insurers.

A Medicare Advantage Plan is a type of Medicare health plan offered by a private company that contracts with Medicare to provide you with all your Part A and Part B benefits but is paid for by the private insurance company rather than Medicare. There are many types of Medicare Advantage programs.

NOTES:
The federal and state governments provide **Medicaid** for those people who cannot afford to pay for medical services. This includes the cost of nursing homes if the person qualifies.

Other types of options used by individuals to pay for the high costs of eldercare include **longterm care insurance, annuities, life insurance** and **reverse mortgages**.

When an elderly person is cared for, you will receive statements from CMS (Centers for Medicare and Medicaid Services), your regional Medicare provider which varies from region to region, your Medicare B insurance provider, and finally from each individual provider or service that needs to be paid separately such as a physician or a therapist if any expenses remain. My suggestion is to wait until all the billing is in before paying for the individual provider's services.

There are many commercial companies who allegedly can help you navigate the complicated Medicare maze. I was not successful in finding a competent company, but in this area, I would think a professional with legal or accounting background would provide the best service.

Legal and Tax Issues

Several steps should be taken to avoid serious litigation at a future time. These include having a **Living Will** or what is sometimes called an **Advanced Directive**. Any institution that you are dealing with will ask the patient to fill out a **DNR (Do Not Resuscitate Form)**, which indicates that the patient does not wish to be artificially kept alive.

Another legal topic centers on the issue of a **Durable Power of Attorney.** There are two parts to this subject: **medical and property.** An attorney or an equivalent legal authority must write up the directive each time the situation changes. The directive determines who is allowed to make decisions on both topics. It's a good idea if you are the child to sign on with your parent in case their decision-making capabilities begin to fail.

Below are some of the other legal issues.

Patients Right's and HIPPA

Every patient is given a copy of these rules, which include a right to privacy. I've never read the statements but in general, they give the patient a right to speak up if they are not being treated appropriately, they spell out the institution's rules on privacy and other policies of the institution. It's a good idea to familiarize yourself with these policies, but often they are complicated and one forgets or is under pressure and doesn't take the time to read them.

Ombudsman

This is a local officer supervised by the Area Agency on Aging who one can go to if an assisted living facility does not adequately care for your loved one. Records of complaints that have been registered are available at the area agency on aging.

Guardianship is a legal designation of care if no one in a family can provide care for an individual. If no one else can take care of the individual, the responsibility goes to the state.

Directive is a legalized statement of how a person wishes to be cared for.

Elder Abuse is any form of harm either physical or emotional that takes advantage of an elderly individual. Eldercarelocator.gov is a good beginning resource.

Elder Law

Elder law is a specialty that takes care of all legal issues that may come up such as elder abuse.

Irrevocable and Non-Irrevocable Trusts and Wills

It's important for the aging person to have in order his will as well as who will be the executor.

The Accountant's Role

It's important to consult a certified public accountant to help you determine what is and is not tax deductible. Some of the areas that accountants can advise you concern tax deductions for medical services, caregiving whether in a facility or at home, and medical equipment. It is also important to know what way to craft an individual's will so that the taxes are minimized.

Social Services

These are often defined as community services that contribute to helping the aging individual maintain as much independence and quality of life as possible. They can be funded by local government or by charities or religious organizations or privately. Some of the services that they provide include aid with securing transportation, dispensing nutritional meals, and providing recreational activities.

Again, the aid can be both private and public.

The Area Agency on Aging is a good beginning resource. This agency is operated by a state, region or county division.

Religious Organizations such as Catholic Charities, Lutheran Family Services and Jewish Family Services are another good resource.

Local media will often have a senior source for locating senior resources and for local senior activities.

Volunteer organizations like Volunteers of America or United Way are another resource.

There are all kinds of Senior Centers and senior programs located within a community through community centers, and churches and synagogues. Best way to find them is to consult your local newspaper or to go online.

Mental and Behavioral Health

In eldercare, **mental and behavioral health** concern the **emotional, psychological** and **social** well being of both the **senior** and the **caregiver**.

The field of eldercare mental and behavioral health is cross-disciplinary. In other words, there is more than one way that the problem can be diagnosed and more than one way that solutions to the problem are pursued and many types of resources available to address both the problem and the solution.

Here again is my "take" on a very complicated topic:

Common Mental Health Problems:
For the **senior**, common mental health problems are depression, isolation, aggression, anxiety, and a sense of hopelessness.

For the **caregiver**, common mental health problems are isolation, frustration, sibling problems, difficult parents, and stress.

Initiation of Service Options may begin in various ways and might include
— Recognition by the caregiver that there is a need for help
— Intervention by a medical facility or a doctor
— Intervention through the senior living facility

Public or Private?
All of these duties can be administered either publicly or privately in a variety of venues such as hospitals, nursing homes, doctors' and therapists' offices. In some cases, patients can qualify for Medicare and Medicaid assistance.

Qualifications
Mental Health Practitioners vary in terms of **education, certification, licensing, accreditation,** and **experience** and also vary from **state to state**. In some states less education is required for practicing some form of mental health intervention.

Scope of work
Some of the responsibilities of mental health practitioners include

— Diagnostic assessment
— Placement of a patient in a program or facility
— Treatment that can take many forms including group therapy, medication, and support groups.
— Research studies and clinical studies

Types of Mental Health Practitioners
— *Psychiatrists* are trained in all disciplines involving mental and behavioral health including the medical, psychological, and social components of mental, emotional, and behavioral disorders. They can be either medical doctors (MD's) or Doctors of Osteopathy (DO's). They can order diagnostic tests, practice psychotherapy, help patients and their families cope with stress and crises. Only psychiatrists can prescribe medications.

— *Psychologists* evaluate, diagnose, treat, and study behavior and mental processes. They must have at least a Bachelor Science or Art degree but can also go onto become a clinical psychologist, which requires a master's degree or a PhD (PhD/PsyD) and two to three years of clinical experience. Clinical psychologists provide psychotherapy, psychological testing, and diagnosis of mental illness.

— *Social Workers* are focused on the welfare of individuals, families, and communities. A social worker must at least have a bachelor's degree.

Clinical social workers provide mental health services for the prevention, diagnosis, and treatment of mental, behavioral, and emotional disorders in individuals, families, and groups. Their goal is to enhance and maintain their patients' physical, psychological, and social function. Clinical social workers must have a master's or Doctorate degree in social work, (MSW, etc.) with an emphasis on clinical experience. They must undergo a supervised clinical field internship and have at least two years of postgraduate supervised clinical social work employment.

A *geriatric social worker* is a professional social worker with expertise working with adults age 65 and over. Often, these are social workers that have graduate level education and field experience in geriatrics, gerontology, aging, or social work with older adults.

NOTES:
Common areas where social workers's skills are employed include facilitating assistance in hospitals and nursing homes, providing advanced assistance in caregiving, becoming involved in senior community services and being a part of end-of-life hospital teams.

— *Psychotherapists* are trained mental health professionals who engage in the treatment of a patient's psychological problems either individually or with others directly involved in the patients' welfare including members of the patient's family. Generally speaking, a licensed psychotherapist obtains a master's degree or doctorate in a chosen mental health field, undergoes a supervised clinical residency, and is licensed, certified, or registered by a government or psychological agency to which they are accountable. In some states, a person with a master's degree in education or psychology may also practice psychotherapy without a license.

— *Other Counseling and Support Services and Mental Health Practitioners* include priests, ministers and rabbis in the spiritual community, psychiatric and geriatrics nurse practitioners, music, art, recreational and behavioral therapists.

NOTES:
The likelihood of an awareness of research and diagnostic studies is greater if the professional has more experience and education.

End of Life

Hospice Care is care that addresses the physical, spiritual, emotional, psychological, social, financial and legal needs of the dying patient and his/her family. This is a concept that refers to enhancing the dying person's quality of life. Hospice care can be given in the home, a special hospice facility or a combination of both. Medicare covers this care for a period of six months or less and the senior must qualify for the care. My hospice team included a director, a physician, three types of nurses, a spiritual counselor and a social worker. Hospice does not pay for room and board.

Palliative Care is a multidisciplinary approach to address physical, emotional, spiritual and social concerns that arise with advanced illness. This care is not restricted to the elderly and is not a specified service under Medicare. This philosophy aims at "comfort care" rather than at aggressive treatment.

Eldercare Policy and Advocacy

There are all kinds of eldercare organizations doing work in the area of eldercare policy and advocacy. Different professional organizations with different interests will collaboratively study and come up with new policy ideas that they wish to promote. A good place to become aware of some of the policies that may be considered is on the website of the National Council on Aging *www.ncoa.org*.

In general, the only regulations for eldercare that are strictly spelled out are in the category of nursing homes. Assisted Living facilities at this point are only loosely regulated and the only avenue for complaints at this point is through the local area on agency's ombudsman program.

Professional organizations and general health care organizations all are involved in defining health care policy and seeking to better the current climate for addressing eldercare needs.

Many lobbying organizations such as the Association of Advanced Retired Persons (AARP) are focused on improving eldercare laws.

NOTES:
Every governmental organization has its own glossary of terms, which may or may not be spelled out for the person seeking information. I have included many terms that overlap depending on the which organization is defining its policies.*

*Some of my main sources included Wikipedia, Eldercareonline glossary, eldercare locator glossary and Medlexicon.

Appendix III

Resources

Yikes!

One can spend hours and hours on the Internet looking for information. Below is my advice on how to navigate the system. It is purely subjective and definitely not comprehensive, but it's my best take on how to handle the maze of eldercare.

How to Begin

Define popular topics and links that will lead you to more resources.

Start with **eldercare.gov, longterm care.gov** or a specific category of eldercare like *senior living* or *home health* or *caregiving*.

Links will take you to all three kinds of resources, i.e. *governmental, non-profit* and *for profit agencies and businesses*. Some links might be *aging parents, eldercare services, eldercare law*, etc.

Every source you consult will have its own list of resources organized in a different manner. Find a source you like and, at least at the beginning, try to stay with that resource for your references.

Reasons for Consulting Resources

1) *General information* such as glossaries or types of professional organizations
2) To find out *rules and regulations* such as how facilities are licensed or what are the qualifications for financial assistance
3) To find out where to go for *financial aid*
4) To find out sources for evaluating and rating *consumer information* such as about a particular service, product, facility or organization.
5) To get *opinions* such as whether or not to sustain end of life procedures
6) To find *emotional support* such as what to do when you can't get along with siblings
7) To seek *legal assistance or advice* on such topics as elderly abuse issues or guardianship or power of attorney assistance
8) To obtain *specific information* on a particular topic such as dementia or respite care or about a particular medical problem like e-coli or uterine tract infections
9) To educate yourself about *current studies* or research being done in a particular field related to eldercare
10) To learn about *advocacy organizations* pursuing changes in policies regarding eldercare concerns
11) To find help for *behavioral problems* such as when your loved one is uncontrollable

The Origins of these Sources

Can be either **private** or **public** and sometimes there is a cross over between the two. The private sources have a variety of approaches to the subject of eldercare based on their own expertise and experiences. The public approach is based more on established data and policy and tries to be unbiased.

Government (.gov)
The federal, state and local levels of government have a myriad of agencies and departments that perform different duties such as licensing, regulating, advocating, making policy on aging, issuing benefits.

Some of the federal and state agencies include the *Administration on Aging*, (aoa.gov) and the *Area Administration on Aging* (aoa.gov), both operated through the federal and state departments of *Health and Human Services*, *Medicare* (medicare.gov) which includes the *Center for Medicare and*

Medicaid (CMS.gov) which rates nursing homes and home health agencies, *The Department of Public Health* (which licenses health facilities), and *The US Treasury* which licenses health care professionals.

Government sources offer information based on rules and regulations that have been passed and put into action by federal, state and regional legislation. *The Older Americans Act of 1965* is the primary basis for these rules and regulations.

There are many new programs such as the PACE program that are being developed at the moment. This is a comprehensive government longterm care program. Your local area on aging will help you find what's available in your area.

Non-Profit (.org, edu)

In the not for profit world, a "mission" determines the scope of the work or the subject. The sources can be informational, they can be advocacy organizations, they can be policy oriented, professionally driven, disease specific or a combination of several different goals. Universities (edu) may often have departments on aging and eldercare that have relationships with various non-profit organizations. In both cases, there is an attempt to be unbiased in dispensing information. Some examples of these types of organizations include:

a) General: National Council on Aging (ncoa.org), American Association of Retired Persons (www.aarp.org), American Society on Aging (www.asaging.org)
b) Disease related: Alzheimer's Association (www.alz.org)
c) Advocacy: American Health Care Association (www.ahca.org), National Council on Aging (ncoa.org), American Association of Retired Persons (www.aarp.org)
d) Professional: American Health Care Association (*www.ahca.org*) Family Caregiver Alliance (*www.caregiver.org*) National Association of Professional Geriatric Care Managers (www.caremanager.org), National Association for Home Care & Hospice (*www.ndsa.org*)
e) Services: Assisted Living Federation of America (www.alfa.org) National Association for Senior Moving (*www.nasmm.org*), National Adult Day Services Association (*www.ndsa.org*)
f) Policy and Research: LeadingAge (www.leadingage.org)
g) Benefits and Financial: www.benefitscheckup.org
h) Religious and Community: Jewish Family Service, Catholic Charities, Volunteers of America, United Way, Meals on Wheels
i) Licensing, Certification, Accreditation and Ratings:

I recommend going on the Internet website of Wikipedia to look up where the various health care practitioners must be licensed. This varies from state to state.

Another good source of information is the Joint Commission on Accreditation of Healthcare Organizations (*www.jcaho*) which many state governments rely on for help in denoting qualifications for both health care professionals and facilities and services.

Finally, various organizations will issue certification for the employees or services that are within their domain. Some of these will be issued by the government (For example, nursing homes and home health services must be certified by the government if they are to receive Medicaid and Medicare funding) whereas other services might be certified by an organization that has developed their own criteria for excellence.

Commercial (.com, net)

In the commercial world, the sources are above all else out to make a profit which means that the entity will make practical alliances in order to create awareness. This can create more efficient help many times but it also can result in taking short cuts that may not be in your best interest.

Like their counterparts in the government and the not for profit world, these companies can be part of a larger agency or they can act independently. Examples of agencies on housing, for example would be *www.aplaceformom.com* and *www.seniorhomes.com*. Individual companies might be specific home health agencies, or caregiver services or medical supplies companies.

Some of the commercial websites offer helpful information on how to choose products and services. The quality of these services varies. Some companies will educate at the same time that they urge you to buy their product or service. It is up to the consumer to decide.

NOTES:

Like all consumer products, there is a huge range of services and products offered, some good, some bad and it's up to the consumer to "Beware."

Also, know that if you sign up for any information, more than likely, the private business will unmercifully continue to try to contact you in every way they can until you block their calls or unsubscribe to their websites. Many of these businesses will also pass on your information to other businesses with whom they have agreements.

Locating Resources

1) **The Internet** including **websites** and **blogs.**

    This information can be *governmental,* (longtermcare.gov, medicare.gov, eldercare locator.gov, *non profit* (aarp.org, ucdavis.edu) or *commercial* (homeinstead.com, a placeformom.com, sunriseliving.com, etc.)

    In addition, it has become quite popular for *individuals* to create their own blog sites. A variety of ordinary people as well as employees and organizations write these blogs. As always it is good to check out the credentials of the person or group authoring the blog.

    Examples of personal blogs but not necessarily recommendations include: *agingparents.com, ecarediary.com, parentgiving.com, caregivers.com* and my own blog, *eldercarediaries.blogspot.com.* The best way to find your way to all sorts of takes and opinions is to start with one topic or website or even "eldercare blogs".

    Frequently non-profits and even the government will have blog sites as well.

2) The **media** including **newspapers, magazines, radio** and **television**.

    More often than not, the media will focus on an individual story or perhaps a new type of approach. Sometimes the media source in a community will form their own resource center. *Caregiving Magazine and AARP Magazine* are two popular magazine examples. A while ago, *Time Magazine* featured a personal article by journalist Joe Klein about taking care of his aging parents. *US News and World Report* for the past five years has published an article in which they rate the best nursing homes in the country. Recently *The New Yorker Magazine* had a feature on a new, more humane approach to dealing with dementia patients that was being tried out in Arizona. In all these cases, it helps to know the research methods and the scope of the investigation. That takes time. Better to go to general reliable sources.

3) **Brochures, handbooks and newsletters** put out by governmental organizations and governmental agencies like the Administration on Aging, not-for-profit organizations such as AARP (American Association for Retired Persons) and private companies such as senior living and insurance companies.

4) **Talks** and **Forums** sponsored by various organizations and companies such as the Alzheimer's Association, community organizations or hospitals.

5) **Books** that can be published either privately or with the assistance of an organization.

Most commonly they will be for profit books that may be endorsed by non profit organizations like AARP or NPR. They can be written by private individuals on a *wide range of subjects*, perhaps just a *memoir* like my book or *informational* about siblings or about caregiving or *humorous* or *subjective* topics. Often they are self-help books which are intended to assist you in weaving through the eldercare maze. Look on Amazon.com and Barnes and Noble websites and you will find titles of all kinds of book titles with all kinds of points of view, some more comprehensive and some more specific. They can be very narrow such as *Eldercare is Making Me Fat*, or irreverent such as *But I Don't Want Eldercare*, or audience specific such as *The Boomers' Eldercare Handbook*.

I purchased three books: *Caring for Your Parents: The Complete Family Guide* by Hugh Delahanty and Elinor Ginzler written by two experts at AARP, *The Complete Eldercare Planner: Where to Start, Which Questions to Ask, and How to Find Help* by Joy Loverde, a consultant in the senior/active adult industry for 30 years and a commentator for NPR, and *A Bittersweet Season: Caring for Our Aging Parents—and Ourselves* written by Jane Gross, a former sportswriter for the New York Times.

6) **Directories** by non-profit organizations like the Better Business Bureau or for profit companies like the Yellow Pages or Angie's List.

7) **Organizations** or **Agencies** which can be either for profit or not for profit

— Organizations that specialize in offering information such as AARP, A Place for Mom.com, senior living.com, Senior Decision (*www.seniors for living.com*).
— Organizations dealing with specific issues such as moving or senior housing are sometimes incomplete or only recommended rather than researched.
— Professional associations such as the National Association of Professional Geriatric Caregivers and National Adult Day Services Association (*www.ndsa.org*). Surprisingly, some really good private companies do not apply to be members of these organizations.

Guidelines for Evaluating Your Sources

1) Rely on the recommendations of people you trust or who think like you do
2) Always go to the source's description of the background of the people who are giving information or performing the service. Look for experience, education and years in business.
3) Find out who endorses the product. For example, when I chose a few general books to help me navigate the system, I chose books by people who were considered experts in their field and who were endorsed by credible organizations like National Public Radio and AARP. Sometimes they were journalists rather than medical professionals.
4) Be wary of how people endorse a product. If the company has a "five star rating," who gave the rating and what criteria did they use? If they have a certain accreditation, who gives it? If they receive an award, who issued the award?
5) Before I buy into a product or service, I like to hear the recommendation come from a couple of different places if possible.
6) After obtaining the initial information, ask questions of a potential service. Keep in mind that the field of eldercare is very competitive. A good way to make sure that the information is good information is to ask the same question to three different services.

www.ingramcontent.com/pod-product-compliance
Lightning Source LLC
Chambersburg PA
CBHW030932180526
45163CB00002B/542